W9-BWS-759

Ear, Nose and Throat Disorders
IN PRIMARY CARE

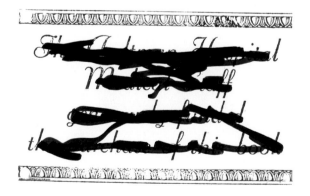

Ear, Nose and Throat Disorders
IN PRIMARY CARE

GAYLE E. WOODSON, M.D.
Professor of Otolaryngology
Department of Otolaryngology
University of Florida
Gainesville, Florida

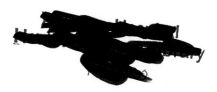

W.B. SAUNDERS COMPANY
A Harcourt Health Sciences Company
PHILADELPHIA   LONDON   NEW YORK   ST. LOUIS   SYDNEY   TORONTO

W.B. SAUNDERS COMPANY
A Harcourt Health Sciences Company

The Curtis Center
Independence Square West
Philadelphia, Pennsylvania 19106

Library of Congress Cataloging-in-Publication Data

Woodson, Gayle E.

    Ear, nose and throat disorders in primary care / Gayle E. Woodson.

    p. ; cm.

    ISBN 0-7216-7431-3

    1. Otolaryngology. 2. Primary care (Medicine) I. Title.
    [DNLM: 1. Otorhinolaryngologic Diseases. 2. Family Practice. 3. Primary Health Care.
    WV 140 W898e 2001]

    RF46.5 .W66 2001

    617.5′1—dc21   00-038811

EAR, NOSE AND THROAT DISORDERS IN PRIMARY CARE   ISBN 0–7216–7431–3

Printed in the United States of America.

Last digit is the print number: 9   8   7   6   5   4   3   2   1

Dedication

To my father, Clinton E. "Woody" Woodson M.D., a family physician for nearly 50 years: He taught me not only to listen to my patients, but also how to let them know that I care.

Contributors

Steven Long, M.D.
Department of Otolaryngology/Head and Neck Surgery
Northwest Permanente
Portland, Oregon
Neck Masses

Michael J. Ruckenstein, M.D., M.Sc., F.R.C.S.C., F.A.C.S.
Department of Otolaryngology
Hospital of the University of Pennsylvania
Philadelphia, Pennsylvania
Hearing Loss, Tinnitus, and Otalgia; Dizziness and Vertigo;
Facial Paralysis

Preface

This textbook is intended to serve as a concise review, update, and reference for primary care providers, as well as an introductory text for students and residents. The upper aerodigestive tract is commonly afflicted by a variety of diseases and disorders. Thus it is not surprising that a large portion of primary care practice is concerned with problems of the nose, throat, sinuses, and ears. Much of the pathology in this region is so routinely encountered that management becomes nearly second nature for the experienced clinician. However, clinical advances are continually developing. Periodic review is essential in order to keep abreast and a convenient reference can be quite valuable to the management of problems that are less frequently encountered, particularly in emergency situations. The first chapter provides a review of head and neck anatomy and function. This information is essential for understanding the pathophysiology of disorders in this region. In some cases, advances in understanding of function have significantly influenced management.

For example, new knowledge on the microarchitecture of the vocal folds has revolutionized the management of hoarseness, both medical and surgical. The second chapter covers special techniques for physical examination of the ears, nose, throat, and neck, including microscopic otoscopy, office endoscopy of the nose, pharynx, and larynx, and fine-needle aspiration cytology for the diagnosis of neck masses. The mid-portion of the book is roughly organized by anatomic site, with chapters devoted to the most commonly presenting symptoms and signs, such as sore throat, nasal obstruction, hearing loss. Each chapter presents the diagnosis and treatment of the most commonly encountered conditions, and provides important information regarding less common problems. The final chapter addresses the management of emergency situations, including epistaxis, upper airway obstruction, and aerodigestive tract foreign bodies. Throughout the book, the focus is on care to be provided at the primary level and indications for specialty referral, also included is information on what happens after the patient is referred. Specialized diagnostic and surgical procedures are described, along with expected outcomes and potential complications. The primary provider and the specialist are partners in care and share responsibility for the welfare of each patient. It is hoped that the information provided in this text will facilitate the communication that is so vital to that partnership.

Gayle E. Woodson, M.D.

Acknowledgments

D r. Douglas Denys, who is both an otolaryngologist and an artist, graciously prepared many original illustrations for this text. His artistic talents and clinical knowledge allowed us to clearly illustrate some potentially confusing concepts. I thank my husband and chairman, Dr. Tom Robbins, for his tolerance and cherished support during the process of generating this book.

Contents

1

INTRODUCTION TO OTOLARYNGOLOGY— HEAD AND NECK SURGERY

Otolaryngology is a regional specialty. It includes both medical and surgical management of problems in the head and neck, including disorders of the face, the ears, the oral cavity and pharynx, the upper respiratory tract, the neck, and even certain intracranial tumors. The term *otorhinolaryngology* is derived from the Greek words for *ear, nose,* and *larynx.* The acronym *ENT* has been commonly used for many years; it is more easily understood than *otorhinolaryngology* by patients, but it does not fully reflect the scope of the discipline.

Before the advent of sulfa drugs and penicillin, otorhinolaryngology was largely the management of suppurative conditions, primarily by establishing drainage. The high risk and grave consequences of secondary infections limited progress in other procedures, such as treatment of deafness, tumors, and congenital deformities. The advent of antibiotics transformed the management of infectious disorders and made it

1

feasible to perform reconstructive surgery in the inherently
contaminated spaces of the upper respiratory tract and ears.
Significant advances have been made in the ability to restore
function and esthetic appearance to head and neck structures.

A large portion of primary care practice is concerned with
problems in the realm of otolaryngology. The primary care
physician recognizes and treats common disorders of the head
and neck, frequently provides the initial management of head
and neck emergencies, and makes appropriate referrals for
specialty management. These responsibilities require a basic
understanding of head and neck anatomy and physiology and
knowledge of current approaches to the management of
disorders of the head and neck.

The Ear

The ear can be divided both functionally and anatomically into
three parts: external, middle, and inner (Fig. 1–1). The middle
ear amplifies sound and compensates for different impedances
of the air and inner ear fluid. The inner ear transforms vibrations
into neural activity.

The External Ear

The external ear is that portion lateral to the tympanic membrane.
It includes the auricle and the external auditory canal. The external
ear protects the eardrum and middle ear and serves as a sound filter
to aid in sound localization.

The auricle consists of elastic cartilage covered with skin. It is
shaped like a shallow bowl, tipped anteriorly. This allows it to collect
sound and also to dampen out sounds coming from any direction other
than anterior. By moving the head and noting when sounds are heard
more clearly, people use the auricles to localize sound. However, the
function of the auricle is not nearly so widely appreciated as is its
cosmetic significance. The normal configuration of the auricle is diffi-

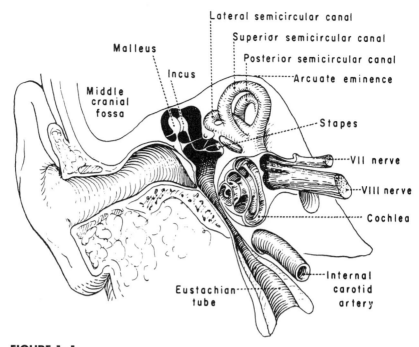

FIGURE 1-1
Components of the ear: external, middle, and inner. (From De Weese DD, Saunders WH. *Textbook of Otolaryngology*, 3rd ed., St. Louis: CV Mosby, 1968.)

cult to describe and even more difficult to create with reconstructive surgery; however, deformities of the auricle are quite easily recognized. For example, children with large, outstanding auricles are often subject to ridicule. Figure 1–2 illustrates the major anatomic landmarks of the human auricle.

The external auditory canal is a skin-lined blind sac that terminates at the tympanic membrane. It would quickly become filled with desquamated debris from the skin but for a unique self-cleaning mechanism. The skin of the external ear normally migrates laterally from the umbo of the malleus in the tympanic membrane to the external auditory meatus (at a rate of 2–3 mm per day). The debris is then shed to the external surface. The external canal can be divided into two portions, the medial bony and lateral cartilaginous segments (Fig. 1–3). The two segments do not form a straight line. The lateral portion points downward, whereas the medial segment curves anteriorly. The skin of the lateral portion of the canal contains cerumen, sebaceous glands, hair follicles and is thicker skin than the skin found in the medial bony segment, which contains no skin appendages at all. The bony canal comprises two thirds of the total length of the external auditory canal in adults, less in infants and children. In fact, the bony canal is essentially nonexistent at birth, gradually developing in childhood.

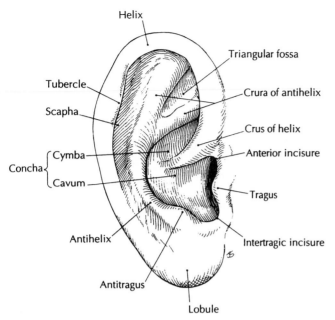

FIGURE 1–2
Anatomic landmarks of the human auricle. (From Bojrab DI, Bruderly TE. External otitis. In Johnson TT, Yu VL [eds.]: *Infectious Diseases and Antimicrobial Therapy of the Ear, Nose and Throat,* Philadelphia: WB Saunders, 1997.)

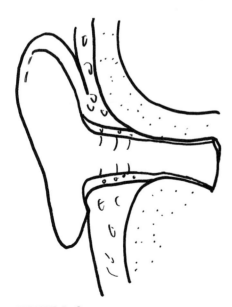

FIGURE 1–3
Segments of the external auditory canal. Lateral canal has thick skin over cartilage with numerous skin appendages: cerumen, sebaceous, glands, and hair follicles. Medial portion of the canal has very thin skin over bone, with no appendages.

The Middle Ear

The middle ear is composed of the tympanic membrane, the air-containing space just medial to it, and the ossicular chain. Normally, the tympanic membrane is an airtight seal, whereas the middle ear space communicates with the nasopharynx via the eustachian tube. The air in the middle ear space is continuously absorbed by blood vessels in the mucosal lining. This results in negative pressure and may ultimately result in transudation of fluid into the space, unless the eustachian tube periodically opens to allow air to enter from the nasopharynx. Only one muscle in the body, the tensor veli palatini, is capable of opening the eustachian tube. This muscle is activated during swallowing.

The function of the middle ear is to amplify sound waves in the air and transmit them to the fluid in the cochlea. This is accomplished by the lever mechanism of the inner ear ossicles and by the fact that the surface area of the tympanic membrane is much larger than that of the oval window leading into the inner ear.

The three ossicles, or tiny bones of the middle ear, are the malleus hammer, incus (anvil), and stapes (stirrup) (Fig. 1–4). The lateral portion of the malleus is imbedded in the tympanic membrane and is normally easily visualized during otoscopy. The stapes covers the oval window. This small bone is frequently visible through the tympanic membrane. The anvil, which connects these two bones, is hidden in the attic, that portion of the middle ear space cephalad to the tympanic membrane. The majority of the tympanic membrane is com-

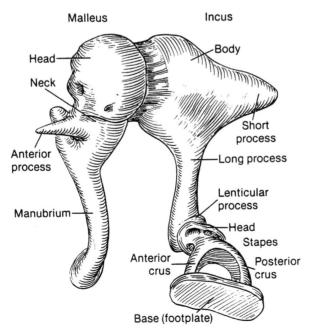

FIGURE 1–4
Middle ear ossicles.

posed of the pars tensa, which has a shallow, conical shape, with its apex pointed medially, at the tip of the malleus. The thickened edge of the tympanic membrane, called the annulus, joins the bony external auditory canal wall. The thinner portion of the tympanic membrane, called the pars flaccida, is superior to the malleus (Fig. 1–5).

The mastoid air cell system is a labyrinth of mucosa-lined air spaces that arise from the middle ear and extend into the temporal bone. The function of the mastoid air cell system is unknown, but development of normal aeration is dependent on normal middle ear function. In patients with chronic ear infection during early childhood, the mastoid bone is dense and sclerotic, with fewer air cells.

The Inner Ear

The inner ear is composed of interconnected fluid-filled spaces encased in bone, including the vestibule, the cochlea, and the semicircular canals (Fig. 1–6). Hair cells in the inner ear convert mechanical energy into neural impulses.

The vestibule, located just medial to the footplate of the stapes, is the antechamber that leads to both the cochlea and the semicircular canals. The vestibule contains two organs of balance, the utricle and the saccule, which sense gravitational force.

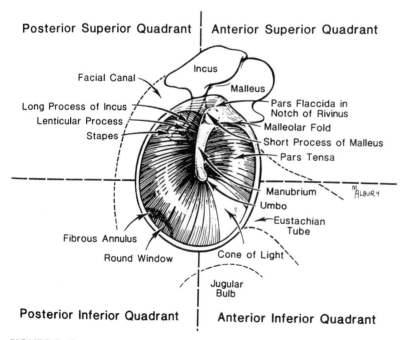

FIGURE 1–5

Anatomic landmarks of the tympanic membrane. (From Meyerhoff WL, Carter JB. Scope of the problem and fundamentals. In Meyerhoff WL [ed.]: *Diagnosis and Management of Hearing Loss*, Philadelphia: WB Saunders, 1984.)

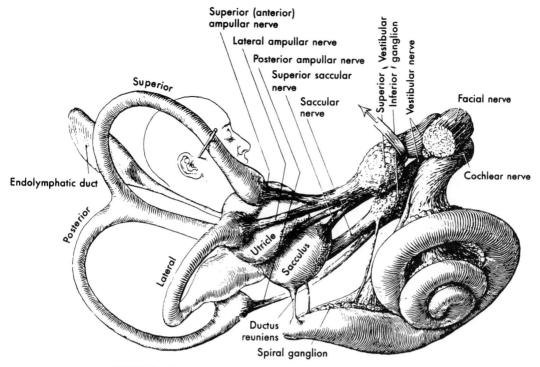

FIGURE 1–6

Inner ear structures. (From Lysakowski A et al. Anatomy of vestibular end organs and neural pathways. In Cummings CW et al. [eds.]: *Otolaryngology, Head and Neck Surgery*, vol. 4, 3rd ed., St. Louis: Mosby-Yearbook, 1998.)

The cochlea is a spiral chamber projecting anterior to the vestibule. It contains the organ of Corti, which transduces sound. Sound waves travel from the stapes through the vestibule, into the cochlea, and out into the middle ear space again via the round window, below the oval window. A watertight/airtight membrane seals the round window. Normal cochlear function requires that both windows transmit sound freely. Bony occlusion of either impairs hearing.

The three semicircular canals project posteriorly from the vestibule. Their function is to detect angular acceleration.

Nerve fibers from the cochlea and vestibular organs make up the cochlear and vestibular divisions of the eighth cranial nerve.

Temporal Bone

The temporal bone forms the lateral skull base. The carotid artery and jugular venous drainage system pass through this bone, and it is intimately related to the dura of the middle and posterior fossa. Medially, it contains the inner ear structures, the cochlea, and vestibular labyrinth. Anteriorly, it articulates with the condyle of the mandible. The mastoid air cell system, which communicates with the middle ear space, is located laterally and posteriorly. The facial nerve passes through the temporal bone en route to the muscles of facial expression. Fracture of the temporal bone may damage any of the structures it contains.

The Nose

The nose is a prominent facial feature and the aperture for optimal breathing. Nasal breathing is highly preferable to oral breathing because the nose serves to warm and humidify inspired air and to conserve heat and moisture during exhalation. The nose also filters inspired air, removing particulate matter. Olfactory receptors in the roof of the nose are responsible for the sense of smell and for much of taste function.

The external nose is composed of a superior bony portion and a cartilaginous caudal portion. The ala nasi muscle dilates the nostril during inspiration. Weakness of lower nasal cartilage leads to nostril collapse during inspiration.

The floor of the nasal cavity is the hard palate (Fig. 1–7). At the posterior limit of the hard palate, the posterior choanae of the nasal cavity open into the nasopharynx. The roof of the nasal cavity is the floor of the anterior cranial fossa. The olfactory mucosa is located here and olfactory nerve fibers project intracranially via perforations in the cribriform plate. Posteriorly, the roof of the nose slants down to become the anterior wall of the sphenoid sinus. The nasal cavity is partitioned by the nasal septum into two chambers, right and left.

The working parts of a nose are turbinates, located on its lateral walls. A turbinate is a bony shelf, covered by highly vascular tissue and projecting into the nasal cavity. There are three and occasionally four turbinates on each side. Turbinates provide a large surface area of nasal mucosa for heat and water exchange. The blood vessels continually engorge or shrink to accommodate to changing atmospheric changes and physiologic demands. For example, in cold, dry weather, the turbinates enlarge, leading to increased nasal resistance and watery secretions. During vigorous exercise, the turbinates shrink, to decrease nasal resistance.

The space between the inferior and middle turbinates is called the middle meatus. This is the space into which the maxillary sinus and most of the ethmoid sinuses drain. The nasolacrimal duct drains into the anterior end of the inferior meatus, just below the inferior turbinate.

The nasal mucosa has a rich blood supply, which is essential to its air-conditioning function. However, the rich blood supply is also responsible for the frequent occurrence of nosebleeds.

Paranasal Sinuses

Paranasal sinuses are mucosa-lined, air-filled cavities that project from the nasal cavity into the facial and cranial bones. There are four

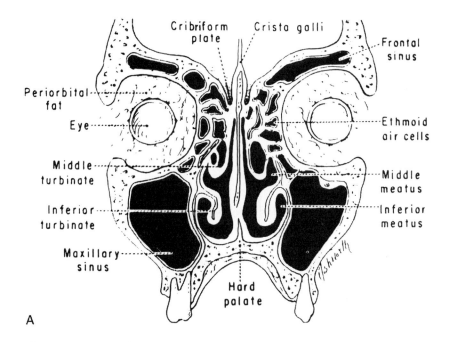

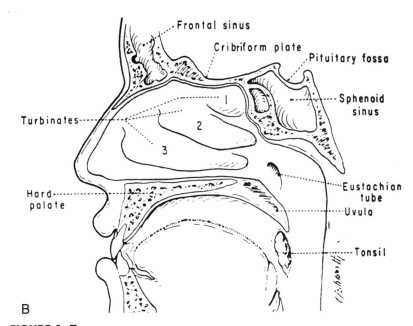

FIGURE 1–7
A, nasal cavity and **B,** sinuses. (From De Weese DD, Saunders WH. *Textbook of Otolaryngology*, 3rd ed., St. Louis: CV Mosby, 1968.)

groups of sinuses (Fig. 1–7). The paired maxillary sinuses are usually the largest. The ethmoid sinuses are variably developed honeycomb systems, primarily in the medial orbital wall. The frontal sinuses extend above the orbital rim, and the sphenoid sinus is behind the nasal cavity, usually surrounding the pituitary gland.

The function of the paranasal sinuses is obscure; however, the sequellae of sinus obstruction are legendary. Sinuses are lined by mucus-secreting epithelium and by cilia, which propel the mucus out of the sinus and into the nose. If the opening becomes obstructed, such as by edema, adverse circumstances may result. Resorption of air in the cavity leads to negative pressure and pain. Impairment of mucus drainage can result in infection.

The Oral Cavity

The oral cavity is the initial food processor of the digestive tract, an organ of articulation in speech, and an alternate respiratory channel. The mouth is responsible for ingesting liquid and solid food and preparing the bolus for orderly transport into the pharynx. Processing of solid food includes biting and chewing, which are complex activities involving coordination among the lips, jaws, tongue, and buccal walls. Oral processing also includes mixing food with saliva. The parotid glands secrete most of the amylase, emptying into the mouth just opposite the upper second molars. Submandibular glands secrete predominantly mucous saliva and empty into the anterior floor of the mouth, on either side of the lingual frenulum. Numerous minor salivary glands are distributed throughout the oral mucosa. The palatine tonsils are located between the folds created by the palatoglossus and palatopharyngeus muscles, at the posterior edge of the oral cavity. Additional tonsil tissue is located just within the pharynx on the base of the tongue. These lingual tonsils are poorly circumscribed and are usually clinically insignificant; however, in some patients, they become enlarged or chronically infected.

The Pharynx

The pharynx is a common aerodigestive tract chamber. It is a roughly tubular structure. The pharynx must serve the conflicting roles of maintaining airway patency during breathing and collapsing completely during swallowing to propel food from the mouth into the esophagus. The pharyngeal constrictor muscles in the posterior and lateral walls form slings that open anteriorly, and these muscles contract to collapse the pharynx. Distention of the pharynx is accomplished by muscles that pull the hyoid and the base of tongue anteriorly.

There are three distinct portions of the pharynx (Fig. 1–8). The nasopharynx extends from the posterior choanae of the nose to the level of the soft palate and contains the adenoids and the orifices of the eustachian tubes. The skull base forms the superior and posterior walls of this segment. A muscular bulge, termed Passavant's ridge, appears in the posterior wall of the pharynx during velopharyngeal closure, as during swallowing. The soft palate approximates this ridge

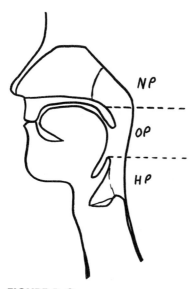

FIGURE 1–8
Divisions of the pharynx. NP, nasal pharynx; OP, oropharynx; HP, hypopharynx.

to seal off the nasopharynx from the oropharynx. The oropharynx extends from Passavant's ridge to the level of the tip of the epiglottis. The oropharnx can be sealed off from the oral cavity by elevation of the tongue base and contraction of the palatoglossus and palatopharyngeus muscles.

The hypopharynx is that portion caudal to the tip of the epiglottis, extending down to the cricopharyngeal constrictor, where the pharynx empties into the esophagus. The hypopharynx contains the base of the tongue and the valleculae and is continuous with the pyriform fossae, mucosal pockets on each side of the larynx (Fig. 1–9). During swallowing, ingested material does not flow directly over the epiglottis but travels around the larynx, via the pyriform fossae, to reach the esophagus. In all nonhuman mammals, the epiglottis interdigitates with the uvula, segmenting the pharynx into a central breathing channel and lateral alimentary passages. In humans, however, the larynx descends into the neck in the first few months of life, so that the epiglottis no longer contacts the uvula. This arrangement results in greater articulatory diversity, which is important for speech; however, it also makes swallowing much more complex, with a greater risk of aspiration of ingested material into the airway.

The Larynx

The larynx is a valve between the trachea and the upper aerodigestive tract. Phylogenetically, the larynx first appeared in lungfish, as a sphincter to prevent water from entering the lungs. With evolution, the larynx acquired the role of a variable resistor, controlling the rate

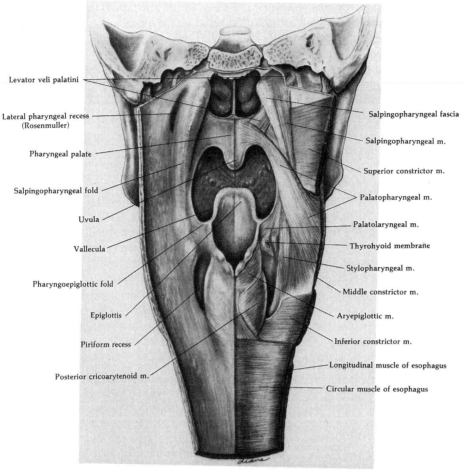

FIGURE 1–9
Pharynx, viewed from posterior. (From Bosma J. Functional anatomy of the upper airway during development. In Mathew DP, Sant'Ambrogio G [eds.], *Respiratory Function of the Upper Airway,* New York: Dekker, 1988.)

of exhalation and dilating during inhalation in response to respiratory demand. The larynx has retained its role as a protector of the trachea, preventing aspiration of secretions or ingested material. It is also essential in generating an effective cough: After deep inspiration, the larynx is closed tightly, expiratory muscles are strongly contracted to build subglottic pressure, and then the glottis is suddenly opened. Without tight glottal closure, it is impossible to build adequate subglottic pressure. Tight glottal closure is also required for a Valsalva's maneuver.

The laryngeal skeleton is composed of the hyoid bone, the shield-shaped thyroid cartilage, and the cricoid cartilage ring. Other skeletal elements include the epiglottic and arytenoid cartilages. The glottis is formed by the true vocal folds (not cords) that stretch between the anterior thyroid cartilage and the arytenoid cartilages (Fig. 1–10) and consists of bands of muscle covered by mucosa. The vocal folds are opened and closed by muscles that move the arytenoid cartilages.

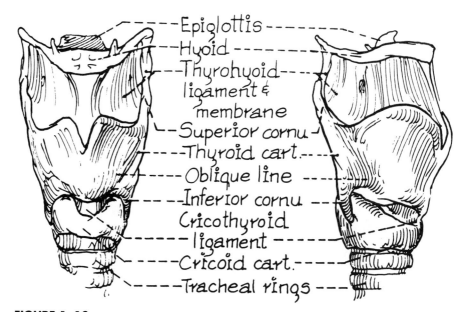

FIGURE 1–10
Skeletal structure of the larynx, saggital and coronal sections. (From Bailey BJ, Biller HF: *Surgery of the Larynx*, Philadelphia: WB Saunders, 1985.)

The vocal folds open for respiration and close for speech and swallowing (Fig. 1–11). The supraglottis contains the epiglottis and false vocal folds. The epiglottis is a leaf-shaped piece of cartilage that is suspended anteriorly from the hyoid bone and projects into the lumen of the hypopharynx. The false vocal folds are bands of tissue just above the true vocal folds. Between the two folds on each side is a space called the ventricle (Fig. 1–10).

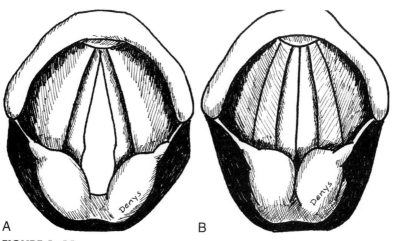

FIGURE 1–11
Glottis, viewed from above in **A,** abduction and **B,** adduction.

The nerve supply to the larynx consists of two major branches of the vagus nerve on each side, the superior and recurrent laryngeal nerves. The superior laryngeal nerve travels rather directly to the larynx from the vagus nerve. It carries motor fibers to the cricothyroid muscle and sensory fibers from the larynx. The recurrent laryngeal nerve exits the vagus in the mediastinum and then ascends in the tracheoesophageal groove. On the right side, the nerve loops around the subclavian artery, and on the left, around the ligamentum arteriosum.

The Salivary Glands

Saliva is important not only for the processing of food but also for maintaining the health of the oral cavity. Inadequate quantity of saliva, due to radiotherapy or salivary gland disease, has been associated with dental disease. There are three pairs of named salivary glands (parotid, submandibular, and sublingual) and numerous minor salivary glands.

The largest are the parotid glands, located on each side of the face, anterior to the mastoid tip and external auditory canal, inferior to the zygomatic arch, and usually superior to the lower border of the mandible. Anteriorly, the parotid gland overlaps the masseter muscle. The parotid duct, called Stenson's duct, enters the oral cavity through the buccal mucosa opposite the upper second molar. Parotid secretion is controlled by parasympathetic afferents that leave the inferior salivary nucleus with the glossopharyngeal nerve and travel via Jacobson's plexus in the middle ear to synapse in the otic ganglion. Post-synaptic fibers travel to the parotid in the auriculotemporal nerve. The facial nerve enters the parotid gland soon after exiting the stylomastoid foramen and then divides into multiple branches within the gland. Surgical removal of the parotid gland is complicated by the tedious dissection required to identify and preserve the facial nerve.

The submandibular glands are located in the upper neck, just below the body of the mandible. The gland is inferior to the mylohyoid muscle but superior to the digastric muscle. Saliva is secreted via Wharton's duct, which enters the floor of the mouth anteriorly, just adjacent to the frenulum of the tongue. Secretory nerve fibers to the submandibular gland leave the brain stem in the facial nerve, exit that nerve at the geniculate ganglion, and then travel through the middle ear via the chorda tympani nerve. This nerve can frequently be seen crossing the posterosuperior edge of the tympanic membrane. The marginal mandibular branch of the facial nerve, which supplies lower lip muscle, travels in the fascia of the lateral surface of the submandibular gland.

The sublingual glands are located submucosaly in the anterior floor of the mouth. Each is drained by between 10 and 12 narrow ducts, which empty either into the submandibular duct or directly into the floor of the mouth.

The minor salivary glands are tiny collections of salivary gland tissue, scattered throughout the mucosa of the oral cavity, nose, pharynx, supraglottis, nose, and sinuses.

The Neck

The anatomy of the neck is complex because it serves as a conduit for between the head and body in multiple organ systems. Diverse vital structures pass through the neck, including the airway, the digestive tract, the spinal cord, and the blood supply to the head. The vertebral column supports the skull. Neck muscles control head position and laryngeal elevation and contribute to motion of the scapula and upper arm.

SUMMARY

Most otolaryngologists cite fascination with the complex anatomy of the head and neck as a major attraction of otolaryngology as a career. The involvement of various organ systems and disease processes results in a diverse patient population in otolaryngology clinics. This also means that diagnosis and treatment is often challenging. Medical management of most common disorders of the head and neck, such as acute otitis media or sinusitis, are clearly within the purview of the primary care physician. Otolaryngology consultation may be required for diagnostic evaluation, possible surgery, management of chronic disorders, or emergency treatment. This book is organized according to anatomic site, presenting diagnosis and treatment of the most commonly encountered conditions and briefly identifying less common problems.

2

EXAMINATION OF THE HEAD AND NECK

INTRODUCTION

Clinical evaluation of patients with disorders of the ears, nose, and throat requires specialized physical examination skills and a clear understanding of the anatomy and function of the head and neck. In addition to observing and palpating skin and surface features, the clinician must inspect and functionally assess interior surfaces and structures of the ears and upper aerodigestive tract. The keys to accomplishing these tasks are adequate illumination and exposure. Devices such as the binocular microscope and the flexible nasopharyngoscope provide a superior visualization of the interior surfaces of the head and neck. Some structures, such as the sinuses, portions of the pharynx, and the middle and inner ear, are not accessible to direct examination. The condition of these structures can often be inferred from a combination of a carefully elicited history and thorough physical examination of adjacent, more visible areas. This chapter covers special techniques for physical examination of the ears, nose, throat, and neck.

The Ear

Complete physical examination of the ear includes inspection of the auricle and external meatus and otoscopic examination of the external auditory canal and tympanic membrane. The middle ear cannot be directly visualized, but much can be deduced from the appearance of the tympanic membrane. Tuning fork tests, or formal audiometry, and clinical assessment of vestibular function are used to evaluate the inner ear.

The auricle, or pinna, is directly accessible for inspection. Physical abnormalities of this structure are uncommon. Disease processes that affect the auricle include skin tumors, perichondritis, and traumatic injuries. Congenital deformities of the external ear, such as microtia or atresia, may be associated with middle ear malformations. Preauricular pits indicate the probable presence of sinus tracts, which may become infected. Infection, congenital atresia, or cysts may compromise patency of the external auditory meatus.

Otoscopy

An otoscope consists of a speculum to dilate and straighten the ear canal, a source of illumination, and an optical system to magnify the image. A speculum is also employed for micro-otoscopy: a hand-held speculum is used to expose the ear structures so that a binocular microscope can be used for inspection.

Proper use of an ear speculum requires an understanding of the anatomy of the external ear canal. There are two distinct segments in this structure, the lateral, cartilaginous canal and the medial, bony portion (Fig. 2–1). The lateral portion is covered by thick skin, which contains hair follicles and cerumen glands. The skin in this segment is durable and can be cleaned and palpated with little or no patient discomfort. By contrast, the medial, bony portion of the canal is covered by very thin, delicate, and sensitive skin. Even gentle manipulation of this portion of the canal can produce significant pain, and minor trauma results in hematoma. There are no cerumen glands in this medial segment; thus, the presence of cerumen in this region indicates that it has been pushed inward. Most often, this is the result of attempts to clean the ear, with a cotton-tipped applicator, or a long fingernail.

The first step in otoscopy is to assess the size of the external auditory meatus and select the largest speculum that will comfortably fit. This provides the optimal lumen for visualization. Furthermore, the lateral cartilaginous portion of the canal is narrower than the bony portion; a sufficiently large speculum will wedge in the lateral segment and not extend into the bony canal (Fig. 2–1). Contact of the speculum with the sensitive and delicate skin in the medial segment is painful and may cause injury.

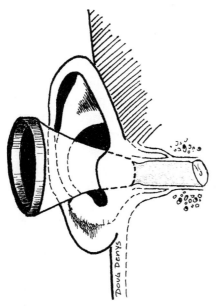

FIGURE 2-1
Proper position of speculum within the ear canal.

The external ear canal is normally curved, which limits the visibility of the eardrum and medial canal. Gentle traction on the auricle will straighten the cartilaginous canal and afford a better view. In adults, the canal curves anteriorly and downward, and the auricle should be pulled superiorly and posteriorly (Fig. 2–2). In infants, the

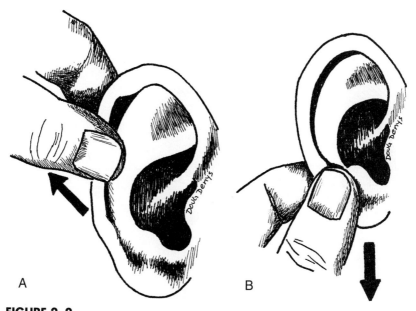

A   B

FIGURE 2-2
Required traction on auricle to straighten ear canal: **A,** adult: superior and posterior; **B,** infant: inferior.

temporal bone has not yet fully developed, and so the bony canal is practically nonexistent. For this reason, the auricle should be pulled inferiorly when one is examining babies.

The external canal is sometimes filled with cerumen or squamous debris or occluded by a foreign body. Such obstructions must be removed to permit complete otoscopic examination. This must be accomplished as precisely and atraumatically as possible. Whenever possible, instrumentation should be confined to the lateral cartilaginous portion of the canal. Most cerumen and foreign bodies are best removed with a curet or wire loop. This is passed just beyond the offending material and then dragged laterally (Fig. 2–3). Purulence and very soft wax require suction removal. Alligator forceps are useful for grasping sheets of dried cerumen or squamous debris but are generally ineffective for other materials. In particular, alligator forceps can be counterproductive in attempts to remove firm, spherical foreign bodies. The forceps traumatize surrounding skin and, when closed, usually propel the object more medially into the ear canal (Fig. 2–3B). *Irrigation is not recommended as a routine method of ear cleaning, unless the clinician is completely certain that the tympanic membrane is intact.* If there is a perforation in the eardrum, irrigation will force water, cerumen, and germs into the middle ear, and this can result in a nasty infection.

Ear canal skin is susceptible to dermatitis (external otitis) and thus may be erythemetous or swollen, sometimes to the point of occlusion. Subcutaneous bony masses (exostoses) may project into the lumen, usually in patients who frequently swim in very cold water.

The tympanic membrane is normally pearly gray, shiny, translucent, and concave. The anterior portion of the tympanic membrane

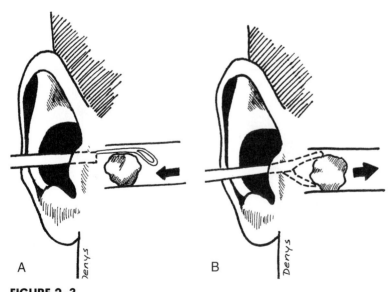

FIGURE 2–3
Technique for removing cerumen or foreign body. **A,** wire loop or curette drags object laterally; **B,** alligator pushes object medially.

is obscured to varying degrees by the curve of the external auditory canal. It is important to inspect as much of the tympanic membrane as possible, and because the entire membrane is not visualized in one otoscopic field, the speculum must be moved around, as the examiner integrates the multiple image into a mental concept of the entire drum, including important landmarks—the annulus and the malleus (Fig. 2–4). The annulus is the fibrous thickening of the eardrum, where it attaches to the canal wall. This is often apparent as an opaque, whitish rim. Sometimes it cannot be discretely observed; still, the junction between the eardrum and canal skin is normally obvious. The malleus is the lateralmost bone of the middle ear and can be seen as a rodlike structure imbedded in the eardrum, extending from the posterosuperior position of the eardrum to its center, the umbo. The orientation of the malleus changes with retraction of the eardrum, with the umbo moving posteriorly. In some patients, the eardrum is so transparent that the joint between the incus and the stapes can be seen. Much is made in many textbooks of the "light reflex," the cone-shaped patch of the otoscope light reflected on the tympanic membrane. However, this physical sign is actually of little or no practical value.

White patches, called tympanosclerosis, are seen in patients with a history of significant middle ear infection. A dull, retracted, and amber-colored drum is often seen in chronic serous otitis. In some patients with serous otitis, the eardrum appears opaque and white,

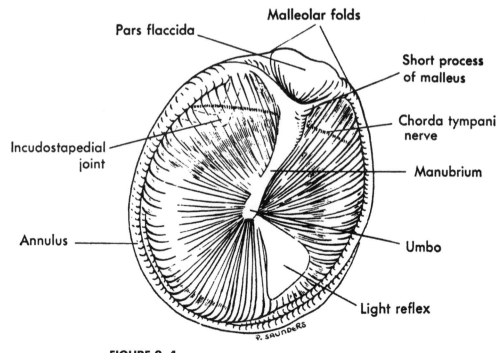

FIGURE 2–4
The tympanic membrane. (From De Weese DD, Saunders WH. *Textbook of Otolaryngology*, 3rd ed., St. Louis: CV Mosby, 1968.)

and blood vessels contrast prominently on the pale surface. A dark blue or purple eardrum indicates blood in the middle ear space (hemotypanum). A red, bulging tympanic membrane indicates acute bacterial otitis media.

The entire membrane should be inspected for possible perforation. If a large perforation is present, then the middle ear mucosa may be visible. Healed perforations are often transparent and may be mistaken for actual holes. These "clear spots" are referred to as "monomers" because the fibrous middle layer of the tympanic membrane is absent. A deep retraction pocket may be difficult to distinguish from a perforation.

It is important to inspect the small portion of the tympanic membrane above the top of the malleus. This is called the pars flaccida, and a retraction pocket or perforation can represent a cholesteatoma, an expanding bag filled with squamous debris.

Pneumatic otoscopy assesses the motion of the drum with changes in the air pressure in the auditory canal. An airtight speculum connected to a rubber bulb is used to expose the tympanic membrane. *Gentle* compression of the bulb increases the pressure in the external canal. If the tympanic membrane is intact and there is air in the middle ear space, the tympanic membrane will move inward. With relaxation of the bulb, canal pressure returns to the atmospheric level and the eardrum returns to resting position. Rapidly alternating *slight* compression and relaxation of the bulb is the most effective means of demonstrating eardrum motion. Pneumatic otoscopy is useful for detecting occult perforations or differentiating between a monomeric area and a perforation. It can also be used to detect the presence of fluid in the middle ear, owing to a useful hydrostatic principle: Gas is compressible but fluid is not.

Eustachian tube function may be assessed by watching the eardrum as the patient swallows during nasal occlusion (Toynbee maneuver). The act of swallowing normally opens the eustachian tube and exposes it to the pressure in the nasopharynx. When the nose is occluded, swallowing generates a negative pressure in the nasopharynx, and when the eustachian tube opens, this negative air pressure is transmitted to the middle ear. Swallowing again, with the nose unconcluded, allows air to reenter the middle ear, restoring the eardrum to a normal position. If the eustachian tube is not functioning normally, the Toynbee maneuver will not affect the tympanic membrane.

Tuning Fork Tests

Assessment of hearing is essential in physical examination of the ear. Audiometry is the most precise means of testing hearing, but in the clinic or at the bedside, tuning fork testing is a valuable means of rapidly assessing hearing. Such tests can be used to grossly assess hearing, but more importantly, they can be used to differentiate between conductive and sensorineural hearing loss. In some cases, tuning fork tests provide information that is complimentary to that obtained by audiometry. A tuning fork with a resonant frequency of 512 Hz is most helpful because this is in the range of speech frequencies. A 256-Hz fork may also be used. A 128-Hz tuning fork should not be used, because this frequency tests vibration, not hearing.

To assess sensitivity level, the examiner should compare his or her own hearing level to that of the patient. This, of course, is useful only when the examiner has normal hearing. Strike the fork gently, hold the tines near the patient's ear, and ask whether the sound is heard. If the patient can hear the sound, hold the fork in that position until the patient can no longer hear the sound. Then the clinician should listen to see if the residual sound is audible. If the clinician can hear sound when the patient cannot, then sensitivity may be assumed to be reduced.

Weber Test. A tuning fork is placed in the center of the top of the head, so that it vibrates the skull and can be heard by bone conduction (Fig. 2–5). The patient is then asked, "Where do you hear the sound?" Normally, the patient will correctly perceive that the sound is in the midline, or in "both ears." With a unilateral conductive hearing loss, the sound will be perceived as louder in the affected ear. In a patient with a unilateral sensorineural loss, the sound is localized to the good ear.

Bing Test. The tuning fork is place on top of the head, as for the Weber test. Then one ear canal is manually occluded. In a patient with normal hearing, the sound appears to move to the occluded ear. In a patient with a bilateral conductive loss, no change will be noted.

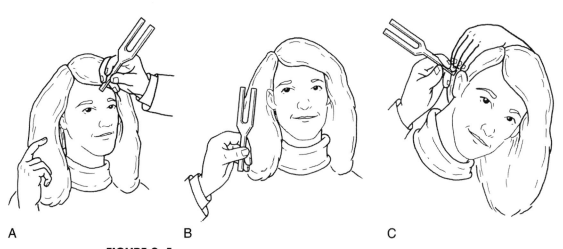

A   B   C

FIGURE 2–5
Tuning fork tests: **A,** Weber test; **B** and **C,** Rinne test. (Redrawn from Meyerhoff L. *Diagnosis and Management of Hearing Loss,* Philadelphia: WB Saunders, 1984. From Roland, PS. History and physical examination. In Meyerhoff WL, Rice DH [eds.], *Otololaryngology—Head and Neck Surgery,* Philadelphia: WB Saunders, 1992.)

Rinne Test. Hearing is assessed in one ear at a time, comparing hearing sensitivity by air and bone conduction. The base of the vibrating fork is placed on the mastoid process, behind the ear (Fig. 2–5). If the patient cannot hear this sound, the fork should be struck more firmly. The fork should be held in position until the patient can no longer hear the sound. Then the fork should be removed from the mastoid process and the tines held in the air just outside the external auditory canal. Normally, a patient will continue to hear the sound by air after it is no longer audible by bone conduction. Sounds are normally perceived more loudly by air conduction, because of the efficiency of the middle ear mechanism.

Although tuning forks are important in clinical diagnosis, a complete assessment of hearing requires audiometry. This is indicated in any patient with chronic hearing loss or with acute loss that cannot be explained by canal occlusion or middle ear infection. It is also an integral part of the evaluation of the patient with vertigo.

Unilateral hearing loss due to serous otitis in an adult may be the presenting symptom of cancer of the nasopharynx, owing to occlusion of the eustachian tube. All such patients should undergo a thorough nasopharyngeal exam and careful palpation of the neck to detect possible metastasis from an occult tumor.

The Nose

External observation of the nose should include checking for any deformities, such deviation, asymmetry, or collapse of the dorsum.

Anterior rhinoscopy is used to examine the interior of the nose. The nostril is inspected via a nasal speculum, to dilate the nostril. The nose is a very narrow space, so a headlight, which nearly follows the line of sight, provides the best illumination. A head mirror may also be used, but considerable practice is required to develop and maintain this skill. The speculum should be opened in a superoinferior, or slightly oblique, axis (Fig. 2–6). It should not be opened horizontally, as this would result in pressure on the septum by one blade of the speculum. Although not dangerous, this is painful for the patient. Anterior rhinoscopy usually discloses the anterior ends of the inferior turbinates and the septum. Topical vasoconstriction permits a somewhat more thorough examination, so that the middle turbinates may also be seen. The best and most complete inception of the nasal cavity can be accomplished using a small rigid endoscope.

Possible abnormalities include swollen turbinates, septal deviation, or intranasal masses, such as tumors or nasal polyps that may compromise nasal patency. A perforation of the nasal septum can cause symptoms of a whistling nose during breathing, epistaxis, and excessive crusting of the nose. A patient with an acute sinus infection can usually be identified by erythemetous swelling of nasal mucosa

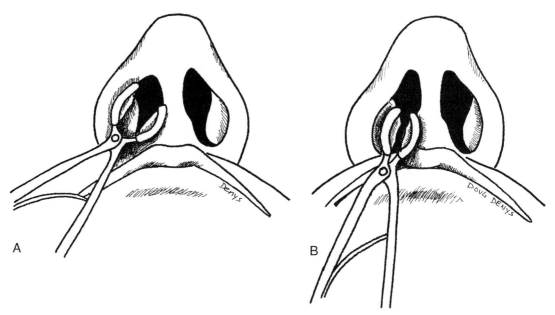

FIGURE 2–6
A, Proper use of nasal speculum. **B,** Improper technique, blade against septum.

and purulent secretions. The physical signs of chronic sinus infection are subtler.

The sense of smell is rarely tested owing to the difficulty of objectively quantifying responses. However, smell testing is important when patients complain of smell impairment or when a complete cranial nerve assessment is indicated. A simple way to assess smell is to present common odors, such as lemon, coffee, and vanilla, and ask the patient to identify the smell. Ammonia fumes will stimulate trigeminial endings and produce a response in the absence of any olfaction; thus, the use of ammonia fumes is helpful for distinguishing true anosmics from malingerers.

The Mouth

Complete examination of the oral cavity is an important means of screening for oral cancer. An adequate light and two tongue blades are required. The term *tongue blade* is preferable to the term *tongue depressor* because the latter suggests that this tool is useful only for pushing the tongue down, to expose the oropharynx. Tongue blades can also be used to systematically expose all teeth and mucosal surfaces in the oral cavity. Dentures should always be removed to expose the alveolar surfaces. Complete examination includes inspection of recesses inferior and posterior to the tongue, inspection of the gingivo-buccal sulci, and bimanual palpation of the tongue and the floor of the mouth.

The Pharynx

The posterior wall of the oropharynx can be visualized easily via the mouth, by depressing the tongue. The oropharynx is only one component of the entire pharyngeal space, which extends from the base of the skull to the lower limits of the pyriform sinuses in the hypopharynx. Inspection of the hypopharynx, larynx, and nasopharynx requires use of either indirect mirror examination or office endoscopy.

Mirror examination is a skill that requires practice. Illumination may be provided by a head mirror or a headlight. Mirrors introduced into the patient should be prewarmed or treated with a defogging agent. A small mirror is used to examine the nasopharynx. The patient should open the mouth as widely as possible and relax the tongue while trying to breathe via the nose. The posterior tongue is depressed as much as possible to provide a space for the mirror above the tongue and beneath the soft palate. Attempted nasal breathing causes the soft palate to relax and drop, providing a view of the nasopharynx. Only a small portion of the nasopharynx can be visualized in the mirror at once; therefore, it must be moved about to show the posterior choanae of the nose, the posterior nasopharyngeal wall, and the eustachian tube orifices (Fig. 2–7).

The hypopharynx is examined with a large mirror. The patient is asked to lean forward slightly, flexing at the hips, with the back

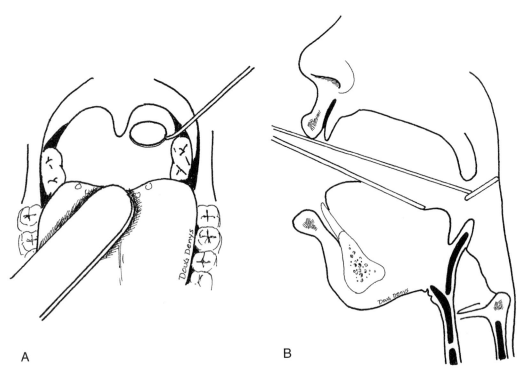

A   B

FIGURE 2–7
Mirror examination of the nasopharynx. **A,** Transoral view. **B,** Saggital cross section.

straight and neck slightly extended (sniff position). The tongue is protruded as far as possible, and the examiner grasps its tip with a gauze sponge. Gentle anterior traction is applied. The patient must voluntarily relax and protrude his tongue. Otherwise, excessive traction (which may be painful) may be required. The mirror is placed against the soft palate and used to push it posteriorly (Fig. 2–8). Normally, firm contact with the palate does not stimulate gagging. The mirror is rotated as necessary for visualization of the base of the tongue valleculae, posterior and lateral pharyngeal walls, pyriform sinus openings, and larynx. At rest, the epiglottis normally overhangs and obscures the glottis. If the patient tries to produce a high-pitched "Eeeee" (actually impossible with the tongue protruded), the epiglottis usually lifts sufficiently to expose the cords. Vocal fold mobility should be assessed by asking the patient to alternately phonate and inspire deeply. The glottis opens with inspiration and closes for phonation (Fig. 2–9).

Mirror examination is frequently not feasible. Some patients have a hyperactive gag reflex. In others, an overhanging epiglottis obscures the view of the glottis. A fiberoptic nasopharyngoscope is very useful in such cases. For patient comfort and easier introduction, the nose should always be decongested with Neo-Synephrine or oxymetazoline prior to passage of the fiberoptic instrument. Patient comfort is maximized if topical lidocaine (4% spray) is also applied. The tip of the

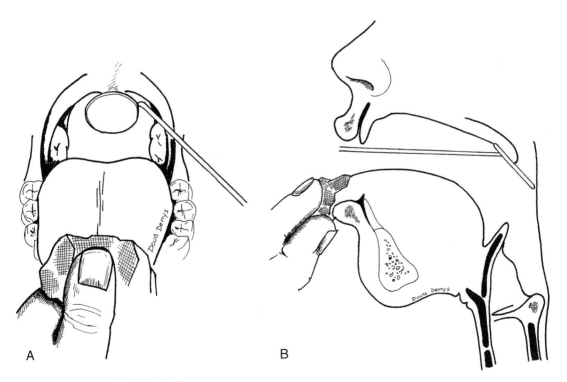

A   B

FIGURE 2–8
Mirror examination of the larynx. Mirror contacts soft palate. Tongue is pulled forward. **A,** Saggital section. **B,** Transoral view.

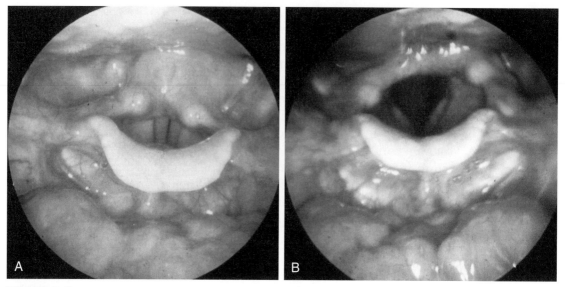

FIGURE 2-9
Structure of the larynx, viewed from above. **A,** Phonation. **B,** Inspiration.

scope should be introduced into the nose under direct vision and then advanced by viewing through the scope. Usually, the best route is along the floor of the nose, medial or inferior to the inferior turbinate. If the middle turbinate is quite large, it may be necessary to pass more superiorly, between the middle and inferior turbinates. The scope should be passed gently and never forced. If there is a spur or deviation of the nasal septum, it may be impossible to pass the scope, and if it is critical to examine the larynx, direct laryngoscopy under general anesthesia may be indicated. At the back of the nasal cavity, the scope should be flexed downward to permit smooth transit into the nasopharynx. During this passage, the patient must be instructed to breathe through the nose so that the palate will relax and open the nasopharyngeal inlet; the scope should never be forced through this sphincter. The tip of the scope is advanced into the hypopharynx, to assess pharyngeal wall motion and laryngeal function during breathing, coughing, talking, and phonation of sustained vowels. The vocal folds should abduct widely with deep inhalation and should close completely during coughing and phonation.

Salivary Glands

The parotid and submandibular glands should be inspected and palpated to detect enlargement, masses, and/or tenderness. The orifices of the parotid and submandibular glands should also be assessed. The parotid duct orifice is usually easily recognized as a small bump on the buccal mucosa, just opposite the second upper molar. Massaging of the parotid gland should express clear fluid. The submandibular ducts open into the anterior floor of the mouth, just on either side of the frenulum. As with the parotid, massage of submandibular glands also expresses saliva, but massage of the submandibular gland should be performed with care because ejection of fluid from the submandibular duct (Wharton's duct) is sometimes forceful and the examiner may be squirted. If saliva cannot be expressed, the ducts should be palpated for possible stones.

Soft Tissues of the Neck

The cervical portion of the head and neck examination includes surface inspection and palpation of deeper structures. Palpation should evaluate the laryngeal skeleton, the thyroid gland, and lymph nodes, and search for abnormal masses. A systematic approach and proper technique will enhance the sensitivity and precision of neck examination.

The first step is to observe neck from the anterior aspect, looking for asymmetry, abnormal masses, distorted landmarks, and skin lesions. Observation of the patient during swallowing is a useful way to assess laryngeal elevation during swallow, and frequently the thyroid gland can be observed as well, as it is pulled upward and forward during a swallow.

To palpate the neck, most head and neck surgeons prefer to stand behind the patient, because this approach facilitates manipulation of the trachea and the sternocleidomastoid muscle. Palpation should be carried out systematically to ensure that no area of the neck is neglected. A useful approach is to begin with palpation of the larynx and trachea, to detect any deviation of these airway structures from the midline and to establish landmarks for locating other structures. The carotid arteries should also be located. Then the soft tissues of each side are assessed systematically, beginning anteriorly under the chin and working posteriorly along the mandible, and then working inferiorly, ending with the supraclavicular fossae, to assess all lymph node groups: anterior, jugular, and posterior. The fingers should probe beneath the sternocleidomastoid muscle. Tissues should be palpated lightly at first, to detect superficial masses and obvious large masses. This should be followed by firmer palpation to assess deeper structures. The exact position and size of any mass should be determined, along with any relationship to the thyroid gland, carotid, or airway. Consistency, mobility, and the presence of pulsations should also be noted.

Palpation of the thyroid gland deserves special attention. It has often been stated that a normal thyroid gland is not palpable; however, an experienced examiner can detect most normal thyroid glands. This is most easily accomplished by palpating while the patient swallows. Anterior palpation, just below the cricoid, will usually detect the isthmus. The lobes should be palpated one at a time, with one hand stabilizing the laryngotracheal complex while the other hand sweeps laterally and posteriorly, reaching deep to the sternocleidomastoid muscle.

Assessment of venous pulsation and auscultation of carotids, although important for evaluating the vascular system, are not considered to be components of the standard head and neck examination. However, when a vascular lesion is suspected, auscultation should be included.

Neurologic Evaluation

When addressing disorders of the ears, nose, and throat, it is essential to evaluate cranial nerve function. There are some special considerations in assessing cranial nerve function in head and neck patients. As mentioned above, olfaction can be informally assessed by presenting common odors, such as coffee or vanilla, and asking the patient to identify them. Standardized objective tests are also available that employ scratch-and-sniff technology. Extraocular eye movements are carefully observed not only for symmetry but also for detection of nystagmus. Testing of trigeminal nerve sensation should always include corneal sensation testing because loss of the blink reflex may be the first sign of a cerebellopontine angle tumor. Facial nerve function is assessed by observing not only the patient's volitional responses to commands but also spontaneous facial expression, such as smiling or laughing. Hearing may be assessed by either tuning fork tests or formal audiometry. Balance function is also tested if the history indicates a possible problem. Balance testing is described in detail in Chapter 4. Assessment of glossopharyngeal and vagus nerve function includes assessment of pharyngeal sensation, as well as symmetry in the motion of the palate motion, pharyngeal muscles, and larynx. Hypoglossal nerve function is best assessed by asking the patient to push the tongue against the buccal mucosa. The examiner can palpate the outside of the patient's cheek during this maneuver to gain accurate appreciation of muscle strength.

3

HEARING LOSS, TINNITUS, AND OTALGIA

• Michael J. Ruckenstein, M.D., M.Sc., F.R.C.S.C., F.A.C.S.

INTRODUCTION

Like many medical disorders, the complaint of hearing loss may invoke a variety of diagnoses, some common and some rare. This chapter proposes a practical approach to the diagnosis of hearing loss that will allow the primary care practitioner to easily and accurately arrive at a diagnosis for the vast majority of patients with this complaint.

A Diagnostic Algorithm

When treating a patient with the complaint of hearing loss, it is possible to simultaneously expedite and increase the accuracy of the diagnostic workup by directing the initial encounter to answer the following two questions:

1. Is the hearing loss acute or chronic?
2. Is the hearing loss conductive (external and or middle ear) or sensorineural (inner ear or auditory nerve)?

Acute Versus Chronic Hearing Loss

Hearing loss that occurs suddenly or evolves over a course of 72 hours is categorized as acute in onset and typically requires urgent medical intervention. Such interventions may include the removal of a foreign body or cerumen or the administration of antibiotics or immunosuppressives. In particular, acute sensorineural hearing loss is a medical emergency that warrants prompt evaluation and institution of therapy (see below). By contrast, chronic hearing loss rarely represents a medical emergency and cannot typically be reversed by the performance of a minor office procedure or by the administration of medications. Thus, patients with chronic hearing loss require a detailed but less urgent workup than do those patients complaining of an acute hearing loss (Table 3–1).

Conductive Versus Sensorineural Hearing Loss

Recall that the primary role of the external and middle ears is to amplify sound and conduct it to the inner ear, from which it is then relayed to the brain via the auditory division of the eighth cranial nerve. Thus, hearing loss caused by pathology in the external or middle ears is referred to as a conductive hearing loss, whereas abnormalities in the inner ear (sensory organ) or auditory nerve will cause a sensorineural hearing loss. The practitioner must be able to distinguish between these two categories of hearing loss at his or her first encounter with the patient, as the treatment of these two types of hearing loss differs dramatically, particularly in cases of acute hearing loss. How can the primary care practitioner distinguish between conductive and sensorineural loss without the aid of an audiogram? The patient's history might provide some clues, and otoscopy is necessary and may be diagnostic, but most important are the results of a simple examination taught to all medical students during their training—the Rinne and Weber tuning fork tests.

Evaluation of the Patient with Hearing Loss

Auditory History

The first priority of the clinician is to determine the time of onset of the hearing loss and whether it is unilateral or bilateral. The following

---

TABLE 3–1 • **COMMON CAUSES OF HEARING LOSS**

	Acute	Chronic
Conductive	Cerumen impaction Otitis externa Acute otitis media Trauma	Chronic otitis media Otosclerosis
Sensorineural	Sudden hearing loss	Noise exposure Presbycusis Genetic Acoustic neuroma

are symptoms typically associated with hearing loss and may help to distinguish between conductive and sensorineural forms (Table 3–2). However, as will be seen, most auditory symptoms can be associated with either form of hearing loss.

Otalgia. In the child, pain in the ear most commonly results from an infectious pathology (otitis externa/media), whereas in the adult it may result from these illnesses or may be associated with attacks of Meniere's disease. However, in the adult, otalgia is most commonly referred from other head and neck sites (see discussion below).

Aural Fullness. A sensation that the ears are plugged or full is most commonly associated with middle ear dysfunction (e.g., otitis media, otosclerosis, eustachian tube dysfunction). However, it also may be associated with sensorineural forms of hearing loss, particularly Meniere's disease. Aural fullness in the absence of hearing loss may be referred from nonauditory sites. For example, dysfunction of the temporomandibular joint or myofascial pain disorders of the head and neck may create a sense of fullness in the ear.

Otorrhea. Purulent discharge from the ear is a sign of an infectious external or middle ear pathology.

Hypercusis and Diplacusis. Hypercusis, a sensation that sounds are overly loud and uncomfortable, and diplacusis, a sensation that the same sound has different pitches (frequencies) in different ears, are symptoms associated with sensorineural hearing loss of inner ear (cochlear) origin.

Paracusis. Words are perceived more clearly in a noisy environment, which is indicative of a conductive (middle ear) hearing loss.

TABLE 3–2 · **AUDITORY HISTORY AS IT RELATES TO THE CAUSE OF THE HEARING LOSS**

	Conductive	Sensorineural
Otalgia (child)	+++	−
Otalgia (adult)	++	+
Otorrhea	+++	−
Aural fullness	+++	+
Hearing fluctuation	++	+
Hypercusis	−	+++
Diplacusis	−	+++
Tinnitus	+	+++
Vertigo	+	+++

Fluctuation in Hearing Intensity. A fluctuation of hearing intensity may indicate a conductive (eustachian tube dysfunction, otitis media) or sensorineural hearing loss. Meniere's disease represents the classic form of fluctuating sensorineural hearing loss, but genetic forms of hearing loss have also been shown to fluctuate.

Tinnitus. Tinnitus is a ubiquitous complaint in patients with and without hearing loss. It is more commonly associated with sensorineural loss but may also be seen in patients with a conductive loss. Tinnitus is discussed in a separate discussion below.

Vertigo. True rotatory vertigo may be associated with inner ear dysfunction and sensorineural hearing loss. A limited past medical history should be sought to investigate the following factors:

- Family history of premature hearing loss. This is associated with a genetic form of sensorineural hearing loss.

- Noise exposure (work and recreational)

- Ototoxin exposure (hospitalization for administration of aminoglycosides or cisplatin, nonsteroidal anti-inflammatory drugs (NSAIDs), furosemide when given in conjunction with other ototoxins, erythromycin (high dose), vancomycin)

- Head trauma (temporal bone trauma)

- Barotrauma (airplane, diving)

- Recurrent episodes of otitis media

- Antecedent viral infection in acute hearing loss

Otoscopy

Evaluation of the external ear canal and tympanic membrane may reveal evidence of cerumen impaction, otitis externa, or otitis media. Pneumatic otoscopy, in which air is blown into the external canal through the otoscope to evaluate tympanic membrane mobility, may be helpful in the diagnosis of otitis media with effusion. A tympanic membrane perforation may be seen in cases of chronic otitis media or ear trauma. It is critical not to "overcall" findings on otoscopy. If an obvious finding such as acute otitis media (AOM) is not present, look for other causes of the hearing loss!

Rinne and Weber Tuning Fork Tests

These examinations, using the 512-Hz tuning fork, are invaluable aids in the workup of hearing loss.

In the Weber test, the tuning fork is held in the middle of the forehead, at the apex of the skull, or between the two upper incisors, and the patient is asked to localize the sound. In a conductive hearing loss, the sound will localize to the ear in which the patient perceives the hearing loss. In a sensorineural loss, the sound is localized to the good ear. It takes only a minimal conductive hearing loss for the Weber to lateralize; therefore, it is the most sensitive of the tuning fork tests.

The Rinne test involves placing the tuning fork firmly on the mastoid tip behind the ear (a measure of bone conduction) and then moving it so that it resonates beside the ear (a measure of air conduction). In conductive hearing loss, the sound is louder when conducted by bone (a negative finding), whereas in normal hearing or sensorineural hearing loss, the air conduction is louder (a positive finding). A 20-dB conductive loss is required for the findings for the Rinne test to be considered negative; therefore, a conductive loss of between 5 and 20 dB will not be detected by the Rinne. One caveat is that in the youngest children, tuning fork tests are unreliable, so the examiner must rely on other measures, such as pneumatic otoscopy, tympanometry, or audiometry. A common complaint of clinicians in training is that although they had learned how to perform tuning fork tests during their basic training, the limited amount of time they were required to use these tests left them unsure of their names, what constituted a positive or negative finding, and what the results meant. The easiest way for clinicians to remind themselves of the meaning of the tests is to excuse themselves from the examining room and quickly perform these tests on themselves. Occluding one ear canal with a finger will cause the Weber to lateralize to the obstructed side (indicative of a conductive loss) and will produce negative findings for the Rinne test. Remembering the names of the tuning fork tests is much less important than knowing what the results from these examinations mean.

The Audiogram

A proper hearing test consists of a basic audiometric test battery ideally administered by a certified audiologist, who is a professional with graduate-level education in auditory testing. The audiogram will identify a hearing loss and its severity, and determine whether the loss is conductive or sensorineural. It also provides information concerning middle ear function and the patient's reliability in reporting hearing quality. It is indicated in all cases of chronic hearing loss and in acute cases of hearing loss where the cause is not obvious (i.e., in cases where evaluation has ruled out cerumen impaction or otitis media).

Common Causes of Acute Hearing Loss

Cerumen Impaction

Cause. Cerumen (earwax) is a naturally produced substance generated by the skin and sebacious and ceruminous glands of the external ear. It functions to coat the external ear, protecting it from invading microorganisms. The ear canal possesses a self-cleansing mechanism of clearing ceruminous debris, via a programmed lateral migration of the material through the canal that results in its extrusion at the meatus. However, accumulations can become impacted in the ear canal, typically when patients attempt to clean their ear canals with cotton swabs. People who wear headphones or hearing aids are also prone to cerumen impaction. Narrow or tortuous ear canals or a genetic failure of the lateral migration mechanism may also cause this disorder.

Presentation. Patients may complain of mild hearing loss or fullness, typically occurring after a shower or a swim, as the wax absorbs water and expands to fill the canal.

Diagnosis and Treatment. Diagnosis is confirmed by visualization of the impaction during otoscopy. The cerumen may be removed by syringe irrigation, curetting, or suction. Syringing an ear is technically easier in an adult than in a child. Prior to syringing an ear, the clinician should make sure there is no history of tympanic membrane perforation. A blunt-tipped syringe designed for ear irrigation should be used and tepid (room-temperature) water should be employed to avoid vertigo induced by a caloric stimulus. The syringe should be directed anteroinferiorly, to accommodate the natural course of the external ear canal. Cerumen lodged in the lateral portion of the canal may also be removed using ear curets, which should be used with the ear canal visualized under direct light, such as that afforded by a head mirror or head lamp. Suction is another effective, atraumatic technique of removal that must be performed under direct visualization with appropriate-size ear microsuctions. Patients with recurrent impaction should be counseled to apply a softening agent (e.g., mineral oil, baby oil, or hydrogen peroxide) for several nights prior to reporting for cerumen removal, as this will facilitate extraction. Referral should be considered in cases in which attempted removal leads to pain, bleeding, or failure to remove the cerumen, or in cases of known tympanic membrane perforation.

Otitis Externa

Cause. Otitis externa is an inflammatory disease of the skin of the external ear that is caused by a bacterial or fungal infection or by an underlying dermatitis. It may occur after swimming in contaminated water (hence the name *swimmer's ear*) and is particularly prevalent in the warm, humid summer months.

Presentation. Bacterial infection (*Staphylococcus, Pseudomonas*) will cause a painful swelling of the external ear canal associated with otorrhea and decreased hearing. Fungal otitis externa presents as a more chronic process, with the primary complaint often being itching. Candidal otitis externa is particularly common in hearing aid users. Infection by *Aspergillus niger* tends to elicit more pain and swelling than is associated with a *Candida* infection. Patients with an underlying dermatitis present with chronic itching and or discharge. The chronic inflammation makes these ears more susceptible to bacterial or fungal superinfection.

Diagnosis. Bacterial otitis externa will cause a painful, swollen ear canal. Gently, pulling back on the auricle or palpating the tragus will elicit pain. Otoscopy must be performed gently, as introducing the speculum into the canal can cause severe pain. Purulent and squamous debris will be visualized on otoscopy. The canal is often too swollen to allow for visualization of the tympanic membrane. Candidal otitis externa will cause itching and occasionally swelling. White hyphae can be visualized on otoscopy. *Aspergillus* species, typically *A. niger,* can cause pain and swelling, but typically less than that found in bacterial infection. Otoscopic inspection of an ear infected with *A. niger* will reveal classic white and black debris resembling wet newspaper. Contact dermatitis causes an erythematous, excoriated ear canal with scaling of the auricle. Culture is not routinely required, as bacterial infections are invariably caused by staphylococcal or pseudomonal species. However, if the infection is persistent, then culturing for bacteria and fungus can be helpful in determining appropriate management.

Natural History. Virtually all infections respond well to therapeutic interventions.

Complications. Bacterial infections can spread to the surrounding soft tissues, causing cellulitis of the auricle and surrounding skin. Chronic dermatitic inflammation can cause scarring and consequent narrowing of the canal. **Malignant otitis externa** represents a necrotizing osteomyelitis of the skull base. It occurs in those who are immunocompromised (e.g., those with diabetes mellitus, leukemia, or human immunodeficiency virus [HIV]). These patients present with persistent otitis externa and progressive cranial nerve palsies, with the facial nerve being the most common nerve involved. Spread of the disease along the skull base can prove fatal.

Treatment. Treatment of bacterial otitis externa consists of gentle cleansing followed by administration of antibacterial–corticosteroid drops (e.g., Cortisporin, Cipro hydrochloride). If the canal is extremely swollen, a cotton or sponge wick may need to be placed in the canal to facilitate administration of drops. In more severe or persistent disease, or if the patient has diabetes mellitus, it may be advisable to add an oral quinolone antibiotic to the treatment regimen.

Infection caused by yeast (e.g., *Candida*). Is best treated with cleansing followed by administration of imidazole drops (e.g., Lotrimin) or by painting the ear canal with a topical dye (e.g., gentian violet). Recurrent yeast infection may be prevented by the application of acidified drops (e.g., 2% acetic acid [Otic-Domeboro or VōSoL HC] 3% boric acid in 70% alcohol). Treatment of *A. niger* can be more difficult and should include meticulous cleansing of the ear followed by either the application of acidified otic drops or painting the ear with gentian violet. Persistent infections may heal subsequent to the administration of oral itraconazole. Chronic dermatitis is best treated with a corticosteroid lotion. Cultures should be taken to rule out superinfection.

Malignant otitis externa requires aggressive medical, and sometimes surgical, intervention. Radiologic studies, including radionuclide and computed tomography (CT) scans are used to confirm the diagnosis. Systemic antipseudomonal antibiotics for an average of 6 weeks are the mainstays of treatment. Surgical intervention is occasionally required for debridement of the infected temporal bone.

When to Refer. Patients with otitis externa that is refractory to the interventions described above should be referred to an otolaryngologist. A multidisciplinary team including specialists in otolaryngology and infectious disease should always manage malignant otitis externa.

Suggested Readings

Bingham BJB, Hawke M, Kwok P. *Atlas of Clinical Otology.* New York: Mosby, 1992.

Bojrab DI, Bruderly T, Abdulrazzak Y. Otitis externa. *Otolaryngol Clin North Am* 29:761–782, 1996.

Hawke M, Jahn AF. *Disease of the Ear.* New York: Gower, 1987.

Mirza N. Otitis externa. Management in the primary care office. *Postgrad Med* 99:153–158, 1996.

Slattery WH III, Brackmann DE. Skull base osteomyelitis. Malignant external otitis. *Otolaryngol Clin North Am* 29:795–806, 1996.

Acute Otitis Media

Cause. Acute otitis media is a bacterial infection of the middle ear space, typically occurring subsequent to an upper respiratory infection (URI) or an exposure to rapid pressure changes (barotrauma, as with airplane descent or diving). It is particularly common in the child but much less common in the adult. Offending organisms most commonly include *Streptococcus pneumoniae, Haemophilus influenzae,* and *Branhamella catarrhalis.*

Presentation. Prior to the availability of antimicrobial therapy, otitis media was documented to progress through a series of stages. In its early stages (hyperemia and exudation), the patient presents with aural fullness that quickly progresses to otalgia, fever, and decreased hearing. Further progression of the disease is considered (see Complications).

Diagnosis. Diagnosis of AOM is based on a history of acute otalgia, fullness, and decreased hearing. As these findings are not specific for AOM, it is critical that they be corroborated by an accurate inspection of the tympanic membrane via otoscopy. In the earliest stage of AOM, the drum will appear dull and vascular injection will occur along the manubrium of the malleus and around the periphery of the tympanic membrane. This will quickly evolve into the exudative phase, in which the drum is red, thickened, and bulging and the landmarks are lost.

Natural History. Left untreated, the infection will progress to the suppurative phase, at which point the drum perforates and a mucopurulent discharge drains into the external ear. Perforation is typically preceded by intense pain that is relieved once the drum perforates. In the majority of patients, the infection resolves after the drum perforates and the infection drains. However, in a significant minority, complications of the infection will develop.

Complications. The mastoid contains a labyrinth of air cells that communicate directly with the middle ear. Any infection of the middle ear, either acute or chronic, will also cause inflammation within the mucosal lining of the mastoid portion of the temporal bone. Thus, a suppurative exudate will be present in the mastoid air cells during an AOM. Although technically this condition could be classified as mastoiditis, it does not represent the clinical disorder commonly referred to as mastoiditis. The medical literature characterizes **acute mastoiditis** as a persistent infection of the middle ear space that is manifested by purulent otorrhea, fever, and tenderness and erythema of the mastoid process. This condition generally does not warrant surgery and is treated with parenteral antibiotics, the choice of which is based on results of culture of the ear discharge. By contrast, when otolaryngologists refer to mastoiditis, they typically refer to **acute coalescent mastoiditis.** This is a suppurative condition in which the bacterial infection causes a breakdown (coalescence) of mastoid air cells, leading to an accumulation of purulent material within these enlarged spaces. It typically takes a minimum of 5 days to develop after the onset of an acute otitis media. It is manifested by persistent purulent otorrhea, fever, and deep pain in the mastoid bone that can be elicited by firm pressure. If the areas of coalescence involve the lateral cortex, subperiosteal abscesses may form on the lateral aspect of the mastoid process (causing a fluctuant postauricular swelling and a protruding ear), at the mastoid tip (Bezold's abscess), and in the region of the zygomatic root. Keep in mind that chronic otorrhea can result in cellulitis of the ear that may mimic subperiosteal abscess. The diagnosis of coalescent mastoiditis can be established only by using radiologic studies. Computed tomography scan of the temporal bone has largely superseded traditional mastoid radiography. Differentiating between mastoiditis with or without coalescence is important, as the treatment of these two entities differs.

Other Complications of Acute Otitis Media. The majority of spontaneous tympanic membrane perforations will heal; however, in a minority of patients, the perforation will persist, creating a condition known as **chronic otitis media** (COM) (see following). Small white plaques within the tympanic membrane represent calcified scars that occur subsequent to inflammation and/or perforation. This is known as **tympanosclerosis** and generally has no functional consequences unless the scarring also involves the middle ear space and forms around the ossicles, restricting their movement and leading to a chronic hearing loss.

Facial paralysis may occur as part of AOM. Spread of infection into the inner ear causes a **suppurative labyrinthitis** that manifests as vertigo and sensorineural hearing loss. A series of intracranial complications of AOM have been described and include **meningitis** (the most common); **epidural, subdural,** and **brain abscesses;** lateral (sigmoid) **sinus thrombophlebitis;** and **otitic hydrocephalus.** All these complications present with fever, headache, neck stiffness, and, in some cases, altered mental status. Differentiating these complications is based on the results of radiologic assessment (CT scan with contrast, magnetic resonance imaging [MRI]). A lumbar puncture is frequently indicated.

Treatment of Acute Otitis Media and Its Complications. The treatment of AOM continues to be controversial and is in a constant state of evolution. The heated debate surrounding the treatment of this disorder concerns the appropriate use of antibiotics. This debate has been prompted, at least in part, by the emergence of multiple resistant strains of bacteria, particularly resistant strains of *Pneumococcus*. At present, most practitioners would treat AOM with the administration of a 7- to 10-day course of oral antibiotics. Amoxicillin, at standard doses (40 mg/kg), is still regarded as the drug of choice for this disorder, provided that there is not a high endemic incidence of penicillin-resistant *Pneumococcus* in the region. Doubling the dose of amoxicillin has been advocated when penicillin-resistant strains of *Pneumococcus* are a diagnostic consideration. An alternative first-line medication in penicillin allergic children is a combination of erythromycin and sulfonamide (Pediazole). Appropriate alternative medications that can be administered when antibiotic resistance is suspected include amoxicillin–clavulanate (Augmentin), a second-generation cephalosporin (e.g., cefuroxime), and, in adults, a quinolone that covers respiratory pathogens (levofloxacin, trovafloxacin, grepafloxacin). The role of later-generation macrolides (clarithromycin, azithromycin) is controversial owing to the emergence of bacterial strains resistant to these drugs. The difficulties posed by antibiotic-resistant bacteria have rekindled interest in tympanocentesis, a procedure in which the middle ear effusion is sampled by a needle passed through the inferior portion of the tympanic membrane and connected to a syringe or an aspirator. The effusion can then be cultured and the appropriate antibiotic choice can be made. Currently, tympanocentesis may be indicated for patients in whom AOM develops while they are taking antibiotics or for those whose AOM fails to respond to antibiotic treatment, in cases of immunocompromise, in AOM in the neonate, or in cases involving a seriously ill child. Over the coming years, the list of indications for tympanocentesis may well be expanded.

Acute mastoiditis without coalescence is treated with drainage of the ear (myringotomy with or without tube insertion) and parenteral antibiotics chosen on the basis of results of bacterial culture. Coalescence is an indication for the performance of a cortical mastoidectomy, a procedure in which the bone of the mastoid is drilled away, thus draining the infected tissue. Mastoidectomy is also performed in cases of subperiosteal abscess formation.

Facial paralysis is treated with ear drainage and systemic antibiotics and may benefit from corticosteroid administration.

Suppurative labyrinthitis is treated in a similar fashion. Intracranial complications are treated with ear drainage and appropriate parenteral antibiotics. Mastoidectomy is indicated in cases of concurrent mastoid coalesence, epidural abscess, and localized sigmoid sinus thrombophlebitis (in which case attempts are made to evacuate the thrombus). Brain abscesses may require neurosurgical intervention.

When to Refer. Patients with persistent infection or complications of AOM would benefit from otolaryngologic evaluation.

Suggested Readings

Block SL. Causative pathogens, antibiotic resistance and therapeutic considerations in acute otitis media. *Pediatr Infect Dis J* 16(4):449–456, 1997.

Bluestone CD. Pathogenesis of otitis media: Role of eustachian tube. *Pediatr Infect Dis J* 15(4):281–291, 1996.

Brook I. Microbiology of common infections in the upper respiratory tract. *Prim Care* 25(3):633–648, 1998.

Chartrand SA, Pong A. Acute otitis media in the 1990s: The impact of antibiotic resistance. *Pediatr Ann* 27(2):86–95, 1998.

Dowell SF, Schwartz B, Phillips WR. Appropriate use of antibiotics for URIs in children: Part I. Otitis media and acute sinusitis. The Pediatric URI Consensus Team. *Am Fam Phys* 58(5):1113–1118, 1123, 1998.

Neely JG. Complications of temporal bone infection. In Cummings CW (ed.): *Otolaryngology, Head and Neck Surgery.* 2nd ed., St. Louis: Mosby, 1993, pp 2840–2864.

Trauma

Blunt injury to the temporal bone (motor vehicle accident, altercation, fall) may cause a hemotympanum, tympanic membrane perforation, or a dislocation of an ossicle leading to a conductive hearing loss. A consultation with an otolaryngologist would be indicated in this situation, once the patient is stable. Barotrauma may cause an acute effusion in the middle ear (see below). Penetrating trauma is usually caused by patients attempting to clean their ears with a cotton swab. Probing the ear canal with a cotton swab may cause a perforation of the eardrum or even damage to the ossicles but more commonly results in a laceration of the ear canal. Management of an ear canal or tympanic membrane laceration is usually expectant, with the patient instructed to avoid letting water enter the ear. However, if the patient is complaining of vertigo as well as hearing loss, an urgent consultation from an otolaryngologist should be obtained, as middle ear exploration will likely be indicated.

Suggested Reading

Kinney SE. Trauma to the middle ear and temporal bone. In Cummings CW (ed.): *Otolaryngology, Head and Neck Surgery.* 3rd ed., St. Louis: Mosby, 1998, pp 3076–3087.

Common Causes of Chronic Conductive Hearing Loss

Otitis Media with Effusion (Serous Otitis Media)

Cause. Otitis media with effusion (OME) is a prevalent condition in children in which fluid accumulates within the middle ear and causes a hearing loss of moderate severity. In adults, this condition typically follows barotrauma or, less commonly, an URI. Despite much research, the cause of OME in the child has yet to be fully elucidated. It does appear to result from a combination of factors, the most important of which appears to be an immature or dysfunctional eustachian tube that fails to adequately control middle ear ventilation and pressure. This allows for the development of a negative pressure within the middle ear, the accumulation of fluid within the middle ear, and a failure to drain infected secretions. The local and systemic immune responses are also important factors.

Presentation. In the child, the condition will typically present as a result of a failed hearing screening or at routine follow-up after AOM. The adult will complain of hearing loss and aural fullness.

Diagnosis. The diagnosis of OME is made by history and otoscopy (which will reveal a dull, retracted tympanic membrane that may be tinged amber). Tuning forks are useful in assessing the older child and adult. Audiometric assessment will demonstrate a conductive hearing loss and a retracted or immobile tympanic membrane. Persistent unilateral OME in the adult should alert the clinician to the possibility of a nasopharyngeal mass and prompt an otolaryngologic examination.

Natural History. In children, OME in 60% of those with the disease will have resolved at 1 month after onset, and 90% recover by 3 months. In those with persistent OME of 3 months or more, the disease is much less likely to resolve spontaneously and intervention is typically advocated (see below). In the adult, the course is more unpredictable and depends on the underlying cause. In patients with no history of underlying middle ear or eustachian tube dysfunction, the spontaneous recovery rate should be high, although these patients might benefit from medical intervention. Adult patients with chronic eustachian tube dysfunction and OME are likely to require surgical intervention (bilateral ventilation tube insertion, see below). In patients with an underlying nasopharyngeal mass, the OME would not likely recover until the underlying process is reversed. If the process is treated with radiotherapy, eustachian tube dysfunction and OME will likely be a lifelong problem.

Treatment. The treatment of OME in the child is somewhat controversial and may include no intervention, the prolonged administration of antibiotics, the insertion of ventilating tubes into the tympanic membrane, and/or the performance of an adenoidectomy. Practitioners are referred to the recent guidelines for the management of OME published by the National Institutes of Health (see Suggested Readings). These guidelines generally call for an observation period of 3 months, during which time the child is followed for resolution of the effusion or recurrence of an acute otitis media. Oral antibiotics may be given during this period to prevent recurrences of acute infections. If acute otitis medias frequently recur, or if the effusion fails to resolve, consideration is given to operative intervention. Myringotomy and ventilation tube insertion allows for drainage of the fluid and prevention of recurrence of negative middle ear pressure. Adenoidectomy is not as successful as tube insertion at the elimination of the effusion, but it has been shown to prevent the recurrence of OME once the tubes have spontaneously fallen out (usually within 6 month to 1 year). Authorities concerned with the emergence of highly resistant strains of bacteria have questioned the use of prophylactic antibiotics at lower doses for prolonged periods of time.

In the adult, OME can usually be cured with a combination of nasal decongestants and autoinsufflation of the middle ear (blowing against a closed nose to "pop" the ear). Although corticosteroids are not currently recommended for the treatment of OME in children, a short course of oral steroids is very helpful in the adult. In persistent cases and, rarely, a ventilation tube must be inserted. A myringotomy without tube insertion can also be performed; however, myringotomy sites heal rapidly and may not remain open for a sufficient period of time to allow for resolution of the underlying disease.

When to Refer. Children with OME should be referred for otolaryngologic assessment when the effusion persists for 3 months or more. Adults with unilateral effusion require otolaryngologic assessment to rule out lesions obstructing the eustachian tube. Adults with bilateral effusion require otolaryngologic assessment if their condition fails to improve after medical intervention.

Suggested Readings

Gates GA. Acute otitis media and otitis media with effusion. In Cummings CW (ed.): *Otolaryngology, Head and Neck Surgery.* 3rd ed., St. Louis: Mosby; 1998, pp 461–477.

Otitis Media with Effusion in Young Children—Clinical Practice Guideline. AHCPR Publication No. 94–0622. Rockville, MD: Office of Health Care Information.

Chronic Suppurative Otitis Media

Presentation and Progression. Chronic otitis media (COM) (or chronic suppurative otitis media) is a condition of persistent bacterial infection of the middle ear with tympanic membrane perforation. Its etiology is similar to that described for OME.

Diagnosis. Patients with COM present with recurrent episodes of purulent otorrhea. Otoscopy will reveal the perforation and, during times of active infection, mucopurulent otorrhea. Audiometric evaluation will reveal any conductive hearing loss, the degree of loss being dependent on the size of the perforation and the degree of scarring within the middle ear.

Natural History. The natural course of this disorder is one of intermittent infection. The frequency and severity of infection is variable and, to some degree, is dependent on the patient's vigilance in keeping the ear dry. During long periods of remission, the drum may heal. In a minority of cases, the active infection will be persistent and prove to be a therapeutic challenge. Patients with COM are subject to the same complications described for AOM.

Treatment. Chronic otitis media can prove to be a difficult condition to treat definitively. The goal of treatment is to provide the patient with a dry ear. Expectations as to remediation of hearing loss are tempered by the degree of damage the chronic infection has caused the middle ear and ossicular chain. Active infections are treated with topical antibiotic drops, with systemic antibiotics added when infections persist. As these ears are typically infected with gram-negative flora, particularly *Pseudomonas,* choice of antibiotics should include an antipseudomonal agent. Surgical repair of the ruptured tympanic membrane (tympanoplasty) is preferably undertaken when the ear is not actively draining. Persistent otorrhea refractory to medical therapy may necessitate the performance of a mastoidectomy, to eliminate diseased mucosa and bone, together with tympanoplasty. Ossiculoplasty, in which the ossicular chain is reconstructed using either natural materials or, more typically, an artificial reconstructive prosthesis, can be done at the time of the original surgical procedure or at a later date.

When to Refer. Patients with COM should be evaluated by an otolaryngologist so that the above-mentioned therapeutic interventions can be considered.

Suggested Reading

Chole RA, Choo MJ. Chronic otitis media, mastoidits, and petrositis. In Cummings CW (ed.): *Otolaryngology, Head and Neck Surgery.* 3rd ed., St. Louis: Mosby, 1998, pp 3026–3046.

Cholesteatoma

Presentation and Progression. Cholesteatoma is a benign skin tumor arising from the tympanic membrane. Its histology is most analogous to a sebaceous cyst. It can arise from a retraction pocket of the tympanic membrane, meaning that a portion of the drum retracts into the middle ear space, creating a epithelium-lined sac. This, a so-called primary acquired cholesteatoma, typically occurs in the superior or posterosuperior portion of the drum. The cause of these retractions is somewhat unclear, although they have been classically attributed to eustachian tube dysfunction.

A secondary acquired cholesteatoma arises when skin from the lateral surface of the drum grows through a preexisting perforation into the middle ear. A congenital cholesteatoma, the rarest form of cholesteatoma, occurs behind an intact tympanic membrane and arises from a congenital rest of epithelium in the middle ear that fails to be resorbed during middle ear development.

Although benign, a cholesteatoma grows locally as keratinous debris collects within it. Because the debris accumulates, it is prone to infection that manifests as purulent otorrhea. Thus, patients with acquired cholesteatomas have a similar presentation to those with COM—that is, recurrent otorrhea and hearing loss. Congenital cholesteatomas often present as an otherwise asymptomatic white mass behind a normal tympanic membrane.

Diagnosis. In acquired cholesteatomas, otoscopy will reveal a collection of white debris in the posterior or posterosuperior aspect of the tympanic membrane. If there is an infection, mucopurulent debris will be present in the ear canal. Audiometric assessment will reveal conductive hearing loss, the degree of which is dependent on the amount of destruction caused by the cholesteatoma. Temporal bone CT scan is helpful in delineating the size of the cholesteatoma and the structures it has encroached on.

Natural History. Cholesteatomas will continue to grow slowly. Chronic infection further augments the invasiveness of this tumor. As it grows, the cholesteatoma will invade surrounding structures, leading to significant complications that include facial paralysis (from facial nerve invasion); sensorineural hearing loss and vertigo from inner ear invasion; and meningitis, intracranial abscess, and sigmoid sinus thrombophlebitis from intracranial extension.

Treatment and When to Refer. Cholesteatomas require surgical treatment, which includes mastoidectomy to expose and eliminate the disease and possibly also tympanoplasty to repair the tympanic membrane and ossiculoplasty to repair the ossicles.

Suggested Readings

Chole RA, Choo MJ. Chronic otitis media, mastoiditis, and petrositis. In Cummings CW (ed.): *Otolaryngology, Head and Neck Surgery,* 3rd ed. St., Louis: Mosby, 1998, pp 3026–3046.
Friedberg J. Congenital cholesteatoma. In Lalwani AK, Grundfast KM (eds.): *Pediatric Otology and Neurotology,* Philadelphia: Lippincott-Raven, 1998, pp 279–294.
Parisier SC, Cohen AJ, Selkin BA, Han JC. Acquired cholesteatoma. In Lalwani AK, Grundfast KM (eds.): *Pediatric Otology and Neurotology,* Philadelphia: Lippincott-Raven, 1998, pp 295–312.

Otosclerosis

Otosclerosis is a genetic condition in which focal areas of the inner ear's bony capsule remodels and hardens. If the otosclerotic focus fixes the stapes, then a conductive hearing loss will ensue. Patients will present in their middle decades of life with progressive hearing loss. In established cases of otosclerosis, otoscopic examination findings are typically normal but tuning forks confirm the presence of a conductive hearing loss. Family history is often positive for this condition. Thus, otosclerosis is strongly suspected in patients with a conductive hearing loss without a history of significant otologic disease and normal findings on otoscopy. Treatment options include a hearing aid or surgical replacement of the diseased stapes with an artificial prosthesis (stapedectomy).

Suggested Readings

House JW. Otosclerosis. In Cummings CW (ed.): *Otolaryngology, Head and Neck Surgery,* St. Louis: Mosby, 1998, pp 3126–3138.
House JW. Otosclerosis. *Otolaryngol Clin North Am* 26:323–503, 1993.

Acute (Sudden) Sensorineural Hearing Loss

Presentation and Progression. Identifiable causes of acute sensorineural hearing loss are usually fairly easily recognized. The patient having undergone an ototoxin exposure (typically intravenous aminoglycosides or cisplatin), a blast-type noise exposure, or a head trauma will present with a straightforward history. Unfortunately, these forms of hearing loss lead to irreversible inner ear pathology. By contrast, sudden idiopathic sensorineural hearing loss represents a medical emergency. The overwhelming clinical evidence is that this condition typically results from a viral infection of the inner ear or auditory nerve. In selected cases (e.g., postcoronary bypass), the cause may be vascular occlusion.

The patient will report a sudden decline in hearing, often noticed on arising in the morning. Associated symptoms may include tinnitus, aural fullness, and vertigo.

Diagnosis. Diagnosis is based on the history described above. Findings on physical examination are normal with the exception of those for the tuning fork test. It is critical that tuning fork tests be performed in the office on any patient with acute onset of hearing loss. Acute sensorineural hearing loss is a medical emergency, requiring the prompt administration of corticosteroids. Tuning fork tests allow the rapid identification of sensorineural loss and prevent the attribution of the loss to a more benign cause (e.g., eustachian tube dysfunction).

Natural History. Overall, approximately 30%–50% of patients will recover at least some of the lost hearing. Older age, the presence of vertigo, severity of the hearing loss, and a high-frequency loss portend for a poorer prognosis.

Treatment and When to Refer. The only treatment proven to be of any therapeutic benefit for sudden sensorineural hearing loss is the administration of oral corticosteroids (e.g., prednisone) according to a schedule analogous to that used in the treatment of asthmatic exacerbations. Treatment must be administered promptly and an urgent referral to an otolaryngologist must be obtained. Recurrence of the hearing loss subsequent to the cessation of steroid therapy may require the administration of the steroids for a more prolonged period (e.g., 1 month). Medications designed to improve cochlear circulation or oxygenation (e.g., niacin, histamine, carbogen gas, high-molecular-weight dextran) are of no proven value in this or any other inner ear disorder. Any patient with an asymmetric sensorineural hearing loss must undergo a workup to rule out the presence of a retrocochlear lesion, such as an acoustic neuroma (see below).

Suggested Reading

Kimmelman CP, Gleich LL. Sudden hearing loss. Self instructional package. American Academy of Otolaryngology, Head and Neck Surgery Foundation, Alexandria, VA, 1993.

Chronic Sensorineural Hearing Loss

Presentation and Progression. Patients with chronic sensorineural hearing loss will present with hearing loss (particularly in noisy environments), distortion of sound, intolerance of loud noise (hypercusis), and tinnitus. By far the most common form of chronic sensorineural hearing loss is **presbycusis,** or hearing loss associated with aging. In the majority of cases, this ubiquitous form of hearing loss preferentially affects the higher frequencies of hearing. Chronic noise exposure (from industrial or recreational exposure) will also result in high-frequency hearing loss, although the hearing around 4 kHz is usually the first affected. Genetic abnormalities may lead to progressive hearing loss that should initially manifest prior to the age of 30. This form of hearing loss may occur as an isolated mutation (nonsyndromic) or together with other abnormalities (syndromic) and is most frequently autosomal recessive. It is important that such individuals be monitored with audiometric evaluation on a regular basis to ensure optimal rehabilitation. Genetic counseling should also be provided. An **acoustic neuroma** is a schwannoma of the vestibular nerve that classically presents with asymmetric sensorineural hearing loss. Imbalance, particularly in the dark, is a frequent complaint associated with these slow-growing tumors, with vertigo being a much rarer complaint. Dysfunction of the fifth cranial nerve (hypesthesia) or—rarely—the seventh cranial nerve (facial paralysis) may also be present. Diagnosis is confirmed with an MRI scan and treatment is typically surgical removal.

Diagnosis. Patients with chronic sensorineural hearing loss will typically have normal findings on physical examination. Diagnosis is made on audiometry. Asymmetric hearing loss warrants the performance of an MRI scan with paramagnetic enhancement to rule out a retrocochlear lesion, such as an acoustic neuroma.

Natural History. Most of the forms of chronic sensorineural hearing loss are slowly progressive and warrant regular audiometric follow-up (every 1–2 years).

Treatment. The mainstay of treatment is hearing amplification with hearing aids and assistive listening devices. Considerable basic science research is currently being dedicated to the development of agents that can protect the ear from ototoxicity. An explosion of research into the molecular genetics of hearing loss offers hope for remediation of this family of diseases. Industry is required to institute hearing surveillance and protection programs when workers are exposed to potentially dangerous levels noise exposure.

When to Refer. Patients complaining of hearing loss should have a formal audiometric assessment performed by a certified audiologist. Unusual results, such as asymmetric hearing loss or mixed conductive and sensorineural loss, warrant referral to an otolaryngologist.

Suggested Readings

Greinwald JH, Smith RJH. Hereditary hearing impairment. In Gates G (ed.): *Current Therapy in Otolaryngology, Head and Neck Surgery,* St. Louis: Mosby, 1998, pp 34–51.

Harris JP, Ruckenstein MJ. Reversible forms of sensorineural hearing loss. In Ballenger JJ, Snow Jr, JB (eds.): *Otorhinolaryngology: Head and Neck Surgery,* 15th ed., Philadelphia: Williams & Wilkins, 1996, pp 1109–1118.

Rybak LP. Ototoxicity. *Otolaryngol Clin North Am* 26:705–915, 1993.

Tinnitus

Tinnitus, defined as hearing sounds that are not generated in the external environment (phantom sounds), is an important medical problem affecting some 40 million Americans. **Pulsatile Tinnitus** (5% of cases), which is typically vascular in origin, may represent a dural arteriovenous malformation, a glomus tumor (paraganglioma) that involves the middle ear, an aberrant or dehiscent carotid artery within the temporal bone, or carotid stenosis. The classic workup for pulsatile tinnitus is a CT scan of the temporal bone and an arteriogram; MRI and magnetic resonance angiography may well prove to be the evaluation measures of choice for this disorder.

Continuous tinnitus (95% of cases) may be cochlear or neural in origin. Fleeting episodes occur in virtually everyone and are not pathologic. Continuous tinnitus is a complaint in most patients with a sensorineural hearing loss and is always more perceptible in a quiet environment. Typical sensations are buzzing, ringing, whooshing, or static. True fluctuations in the intensity of the tinnitus occur in Meniere's disease, in which exacerbations are typically reported as roaring.

Jastreboff and Hazell deserve much credit for reorienting the way clinicians think about and treat tinnitus (see Suggested Reading). They emphasized that although many people have chronic tinnitus, a relatively small minority of patients (10%) are troubled by it. Those patients who find tinnitus troubling do so not because their tinnitus signal possesses unique or unusual properties but rather because their central nervous systems have failed to adapt to a chronic stimulus. Thus, treatment should be addressed not at eliminating the tinnitus signal but rather at promoting central adaptation. A proper tinnitus treatment program should incorporate a variety of strategies that promote central adaptation, including counseling, psychologic relaxation and distraction techniques (e.g., biofeedback), tinnitus masking devices and hearing aids, and, when indicated, medications. Anxiolytics and tricyclic antidepressants have been proven useful in subpopulations of patients who demonstrate chronic anxiety or depressive disorders.

Suggested Reading

Jastreboff PJ, Hazell JWP. A neurophysiological approach to tinnitus: Clinical implications. *Br J Audiol* 27:7–17, 1993.

Otalgia

Pain occurring in the ear or in the region of the ear is a common complaint in both adults and children. In the child, such pain is most commonly due to otitis media, although it sometimes may be referred from the oral cavity or pharynx because of the eruption of upper molars or pharyngitis. In the adult, otalgia is rarely caused by otologic pathology and is most commonly referred from sites with which it shares its sensory innervation. A useful diagnostic aid to help localize the site of pathology is to ask the patient to use one finger to point to the site of maximal pain. This strategy can be used to identify the origin of the pain, which typically emanates from one of the following sites.

The Temporomandibular Joint. Dysfunction of the temporomandibular joint is probably the most common cause of otalgia, typically maximal in the preauricular region. This diagnosis should be suspected in patients with malocclusion, pain with chewing, or a history of bruxism. Physical examination may reveal point tenderness, which reproduces the patient's pain at the condyle and malocclusion. Acute treatment consists of a NSAID and a soft diet. Persistent pain will require consultation with an oral surgeon for construction of a bite block or for surgical intervention.

Teeth. Caries, root abscesses, and erupting upper molars will all cause referred otalgia, typically referred to the deeper portions of the ear canal. Physical examination may reveal pain on tapping of the offending teeth.

Pharynx, Larynx. Inflammation or neoplasm involving these structures will produce otalgia that is typically unilateral and referred to the deeper portion of the ear canal. Any patient with persistent otalgia, particularly if they have a history of smoking and alcohol intake, should be referred to an otolaryngologist for evaluation of the upper respiratory tract to rule out carcinoma.

Cervical Spine. Patients with degenerative disc disease or other forms of cervical root entrapment may experience pain referred to the postauricular region.

Visual Dysfunction. Patients who wear ill-fitting glasses that press on their mastoid bones will complain of pain in this area that they sometimes refer to as ear pain. This simple diagnosis should not be overlooked.

DIZZINESS AND VERTIGO

• Michael J. Ruckenstein, M.D., M.Sc., F.R.C.S.C., F.A.C.S.

It is rare to find a primary care practitioner who does not approach the patient with a primary complaint of dizziness with a certain degree of trepidation. This angst on the part of the clinician is well justified, as the differential diagnosis involves multiple organ systems and a wide variety of disorders. Symptoms that a patient describes as dizziness may reflect ear dysfunction, vascular insufficiency, neurologic dysfunction, or psychological problems. The primary goal of this chapter is to provide a rational, straightforward, and cost-effective approach to the diagnosis of patients with the complaint of dizziness. Following the diagnostic algorithm in Table 4–1 will allow the clinician to establish a diagnosis, implement a treatment plan, and determine the urgency with which this plan must be followed. This approach will be useful to clinicians in both urgent care (Table 4–2) and primary care settings. The latter portion of the chapter deals with details related to management of dizziness due to specific vestibular disorders.

Suggested Readings

Baloh RW. Approach to the evaluation of the dizzy patient. *Otolaryngol Head Neck Surg* 112:3–7, 1995.
Ruckenstein MJ. A practical approach to dizziness. *Postgrad Med* 97:70–81, 1995.

Differential Diagnosis

1. **Define what the patient means by *dizzy*. Does the patient have true vertigo?** Dizziness is a subjective symptom and can represent very different sensations to different people. The clinician must be painstaking in eliciting the specific symptoms experienced by the patient. Defining the specific sensation of dizziness is

TABLE 4-1 • **DIAGNOSTIC ALGORITHM**

1. Is it vertigo? Define symptoms:
   I. Presyncope on arising
   II. Imbalance
   III. Vague lightheadedness
   IV. Vertigo: illusion of movement
2. Is the vertigo central or peripheral in origin?
   I. Central vertigo
   II. Peripheral vertigo
3. How long do the episodes of vertigo last?
   I. Episodes lasting seconds
   II. Episodes lasting minutes
   III. Episodes lasting hours
   IV. Episodes lasting for days to weeks

the most critical component of the diagnostic workup and clinicians must not move on to further steps unless they are confident that they understand the specific nature of the patient's complaint. When questioned as to the specific sensations that characterize their dizziness, patients typically define one of the following four complaints.

I. **Lightheadedness and imbalance:** The patient may describe lightheadedness and imbalance, typically elicited when assuming an upright posture. This common complaint of presyncope is usually attributable to cerebral hypoperfusion when the patient arises from a sitting or supine position. It is typically worse in the morning, after a prolonged period of bed rest. An important point is that the patient does not complain of the symptoms when he or she assumes a supine position. This disorder results from an inability to maintain an appropriate cardiovascular response to changes in posture and/or a stenotic lesion within the cerebral circulation that limits blood flow.

Suggested Reading

Mathias CJ. Orthostatic hypotension: Causes, mechanisms, and influencing factors. *Neurology* 45:S6–S11, 1995.

TABLE 4-2 • **INDICATIONS FOR URGENT ATTENTION**

Urgent care is more likely to be required in patients with dizziness or vertigo with
- Associated signs of central nervous system dysfunction
- Acute vertigo subsequent to trauma
- Vertigo associated with acute or chronic otitis media

II. **Peripheral vertigo:** In contrast to vertigo of central origin, vertigo originating from dysfunction of the inner ear or eighth cranial nerve has few associated symptoms, which, when present, typically relate to auditory dysfunction. Thus, peripheral vertiginous disorders are best classified not on the basis of their associated symptoms but rather on the duration of the individual vertiginous episodes.

3. **How long do the episodes of vertigo last?** Establishing the duration of actual vertigo, as distinct from constitutional symptoms associated with the event (e.g., nausea, fatigue) is critical to establishing the diagnosis of peripheral vertigo.

   I. **Episodes lasting seconds:** Benign positional vertigo (BPV) causes episodes of vertigo lasting for seconds (up to 1 minute) that are caused by a rapid head movement in a nonaxial plane (e.g., rolling over in bed, looking up rapidly). As soon as the patient steadies himself or herself, the vertigo resolves. Benign positional vertigo is the most common of the peripheral vestibular disorders. It is typically idiopathic but may occur as a result of head trauma or subsequent to a vestibular neuronitis or labyrinthitis (see below). Current evidence suggests that it results from the accumulation of organic debris (canaliths) within one of the semicircular canals of the inner ear, typically the posterior canal.

Suggested Reading

Brandt T, Steddin S. Current view of the mechanism of benign paroxysmal positioning vertigo: Cupulolithiasis or canalolithiasis? *J Vestib Res* 3:373–382, 1993.

   II. **Episodes lasting minutes:** There are no peripheral vestibular disorders that cause episodes of vertigo lasting for minutes. The only disorder that typically causes vertigo lasting for this duration is vertebrobasilar insufficiency. The symptoms associated with disorder were discussed above. The presence of vertigo lasting for minutes with associated central neurologic symptoms should prompt the evaluation of the posterior fossa circulation, typically with an arteriogram.

   III. **Episodes lasting hours:** Two disorders cause episodes of vertigo lasting for hours. The presence or absence of auditory dysfunction differentiates these entities.

   Episodes of vertigo lasting for hours associated with fluctuating and progressive sensorineural hearing loss and with tinnitus comprise the classic triad of symptoms that defines the clinical entity known as Meniere's disease. Aural fullness or pressure is a frequently associated symptom. Meniere's disease is an idiopathic disorder that typically occurs in patients between 30 and 60 years of age. It ultimately affects both ears in 45% of patients. Theories related to the pathogenesis of Meniere's disease are controversial and have classically attributed this disorder to the overaccumulation of fluid within the inner ear (endolymphatic hydrops). Although more recent analyses have brought into serious question the validity of the relationship of endolymphatic hydrops to the symptoms associated with Meniere's disease, the pathogenesis of this intriguing disorder remains unclear.

The diagnosis of Meniere's disease is strongly suggested by history. The typical course of Meniere's disease is clusters of vertiginous episodes separated by remission. During the vertiginous episodes, hearing loss and tinnitus will typically be exacerbated. In most patients, the disease will "burn out," leaving them with chronic moderate to severe hearing loss, tinnitus, and imbalance, particularly in the dark.

Suggested Readings

Green JD Jr, Blum DJ, Harner SG. Longitudinal followup of patients with Meniere's disease. *Otolaryngol Head Neck Surg* 104:783–788, 1991.
Ruckenstein MJ, Harrison RV. Cochlear pathophysiology in Meniere's disease, a critical appraisal. In Harris JP, (ed.): *Meniere's Disease.* The Hague: Kugler, 1998, pp 155–162.
Schessel DA, Nedzelski JM. Meniere's disease and other peripheral vestibular disorders. In Cummings CW, (ed.): *Otolaryngology, Head and Neck Surgery.* 2nd ed. St. Louis: Mosby, 1993, pp 3152–3176.

Vertigo lasting for hours in the absence of significant auditory symptoms is most commonly migrainous in origin. A small percentage of patients presenting with these symptoms will develop Meniere's disease, with the full symptom complex appearing within 1–2 years after the onset of the vertigo. A similarly small percentage of these patients will have no history of migraines and will never develop Meniere's disease. This idiopathic entity is best referred to as **recurrent vestibulopathy**.

Suggested Readings

Cutrer FM, Baloh RW. Migraine-associated dizziness. *Headache* 32:300–304, 1992.
Leliever WC, Barber HO. Recurrent vestibulopathy. *Laryngoscope* 91:1–6, 1981.
Rassekh CH, Harker LA. The prevalence of migraine in Meniere's disease. *Laryngoscope* 102:135–138, 1992.

IV. **Episodes lasting for days to weeks: Vestibular neuronitis** is a common and frightening disorder that often precipitates a visit to the hospital emergency department. It characterized by an acute onset of vertigo, associated with nausea and vomiting, but no symptoms of auditory or central nervous system dysfunction. The lack of associated symptoms, the absence of dysdiadochokinesia, and the fact that this is *not* a recurrent condition are critical aspects of the history and examination that help the clinician differentiate this relatively benign disorder from other neurovestibular disorders. Vestibular neuronitis is thought to result from a viral infection of the vestibular component of the eighth cranial nerve.

Suggested Reading

Nadol JB Jr. Vestibular neuritis. *Otolaryngol Head Neck Surg* 112:162–172, 1995.

Physical Examination

Readers will note that the above discussion pertaining to the diagnosis of dizziness and vertigo focuses heavily on the patient's history, with the occasional reference to pertinent findings on physical examination. This focus is deliberate to emphasize that the patient history is far and away the most important factor in diagnosing these disorders. After taking the medical history, the clinician should have a very good idea as to the nature of the diagnosis and should use the physical examination to confirm his or her hypothesis. With this fact acknowledged, the following are the components of the neuro-otologic examination that may prove helpful in confirming the diagnosis.

Neuro-otologic Examination

Otoscopy. Although otoscopy is a basic component of the neuro-otologic examination, remember that middle ear disorders, especially otitis media, only rarely cause dizziness or vertigo.

Tuning Fork Tests. Tuning fork tests are very useful in establishing the presence of asymmetric hearing loss, as is seen in Meniere's disease and acoustic neuromas.

Eye Movements. Abnormalities in the performance of smooth pursuit and saccadic eye movements may indicate the presence of central pathology.

Tests of Balance. Abnormal findings on Romberg's test are fairly nonspecific indicators of central nervous system pathology. Poor performances on tandem (heel-to-toe) gait testing with eyes open and closed indicates posterior fossa dysfunction, whereas poor performance only when eyes are closed may indicate a peripheral vestibular loss. Similarly, patients with a peripheral vestibular loss may fall to that side when given a tandem Romberg's test (feet heel-to-toe, eyes closed) or Fukuda's stepping test (marching in place with eyes closed and arms folded across the chest).

As noted above, patients who have had a cerebellar stroke will have particular difficulties with rapid alternating supination and pronation of the hands and may perform finger-to-nose testing poorly (dysdiadochokinesia).

Dix–Hallpike Maneuver. The presence of active BPV can be confirmed by the performance of a Dix–Hallpike (or Barany) maneuver. This maneuver consists of moving the patient from a sitting to supine position with the head turned and hanging over the head of the bed so the affected ear faces the ground. The elicitation of vertigo and nystagmus with the patient in the head-hanging position confirms the diagnosis of BPV.

Hyperventilation. Reproduction of the patient's symptoms with hyperventilation has been associated with psychogenic dizziness. However, this maneuver will also exacerbate dysautonomias and may also produce nystagmus and vertigo in patients with a known peripheral vestibular loss. Thus, the results of this test must be correlated with the patient history.

Eliciting Nystagmus. It is very common for a neuro-otologist to field questions pertaining to the understanding of nystagmus. To the experienced observer, the presence of spontaneous, gaze-evoked, or positional nystagmus can be a valuable clue as to the site of dysfunction. However, to the inexperienced observer, attempts to observe and then classify nystagmus will likely prove frustrating and uninformative. There are simply too many important factors to remember and too little time to observe the finding. There are two situations, however, in which the presence of nystagmus may provide the primary care practitioner with important diagnostic clues. Nystagmus induced during the Dix–Hallpike maneuver, particularly when accompanied by symptoms of vertigo, will confirm the diagnosis of BPV. The differentiation of vestibular neuronitis from a central event in the patient with acute vertigo may be facilitated by the observation of fixation suppression of nystagmus. These patients will frequently demonstrate very obvious spontaneous nystagmus. In vestibular neuronitis, the nystagmus will suppress with visual fixation on an object and the patient's symptoms will seem to lessen somewhat. In the case of a cerebellar stroke, visual fixation should not alter the nystagmus. For those readers interested in pursuing the topic of nystagmus, there is a very cogent discussion in the text authored by Baloh and Honrubia.

Suggested Reading

Baloh RW, Honrubia V. *Clinical Neurophysiology of the Vestibular System*. 2nd ed., Philadelphia: F.A. Davis, 1990, pp 133–148.

What Diagnostic Tests Might Be Considered?

A basic battery of audiometric tests is indicated in any patient whose history and physical examination are suggestive of hearing loss. Electronystagmography (ENG) is a battery of tests that measures eye movements in response to visual and vestibular (warm- and cold-water caloric irrigations of the ear) stimuli. Patterns of eye movements may indicate central or peripheral dysfunction. In addition, a diminished response to caloric irrigations may indicate the presence of a peripheral vestibular loss, as is seen in Meniere's disease. The tests involved in ENG are most useful in chronic peripheral vestibular disorders, as they provide information regarding the degree and progression of a peripheral vestibular deficit and the side affected. In cases with medicolegal implications and in patients with psychogenic dizziness that requires reassurance that no organic disease is present, ENG provides objective data. It also aids in establishing a diagnosis in patients with an atypical history and in monitoring the response to certain therapeutic interventions. Although it can provide some information regarding the presence of central disease, a MRI scan will typically provide more direct and specific information. A MRI scan is thus indicated when results of the clinical evaluation point to central disease.

Management of Specific Diagnoses

Dysautonomia

Dysautonomias, which prevent an appropriate cardiovascular response to changes in posture, are an important cause of dizziness and most commonly occur secondary to the administration of antihypertensive or antiarrhythmic therapy. Diabetes mellitus, another important cause for this disorder, frequently coexists with cardiovascular disease. Primary dysautonomias are rare (e.g., Shy–Drager syndrome) and are indicated by multisystemic autonomic dysfunction. Diagnosis of this form of dizziness is usually straightforward. Symptoms should occur only when arising, typically in a patient with a history of cardiovascular disease and/or diabetes mellitus. Bedside examination may confirm orthostatic hypotension; however, the inability to document this physical finding should not rule out this diagnosis if the patient's medical history is highly suggestive. Frequently, autonomic function testing using a tilt table will elicit symptoms accompanied by a drop in blood pressure that cannot be demonstrated at bedside.

Treatment of this disorder may be as simple as advising the patient to arise slowly, wear support hose, or increase his or her salt intake. Altering medications or adjusting their doses may also prove to be beneficial. Under certain circumstances, pharmacotherapy, including sympathomimetics or mineralocorticoid agonists, may prove beneficial.

Suggested Reading

Robertson D, Davis TL. Recent advances in the treatment of orthostatic hypotension. *Neurology* 45:S26–S32, 1995.

Benign Positional Vertigo

The prognosis for recovery from benign positional vertigo (BPV) is excellent. The natural course of BPV is for it to remit spontaneously. However, the duration of the symptomatic period is variable, and symptoms may persist for months. During this time, the patient may be quite incapacitated owing to the recurrent episodes of vertigo and the fear associated with these unpredictable attacks. Recently, a very benign and simple treatment strategy has been developed that incorporates positional maneuvers performed at the bedside to cause the canaliths to fall out of the semicircular canal and into the labyrinthine vestibule, where they cause no adverse effects. In North America, the Epley canalith repositioning maneuver has proven to be an effective rapid treatment for these symptoms, eliminating the vertigo in over 90% to 95% of cases and allowing the patient to resume a normal lifestyle. It should be noted that BPV is a recurrent condition and that although these maneuvers do eliminate the acute episodes, they do not prevent recurrence of symptoms.

Suggested Reading

Epley JM. Positional vertigo related to semicircular canalithiasis. *Otolaryngol Head Neck Surg* 112:154–161, 1995.

Meniere's Disease

The treatment of Meniere's disease is highly controversial. A comprehensive discussion of this subject is well beyond the scope of this book, but the primary care physician should know the following basic points about the management of this disorder. Meniere's disease has an extraordinarily high, short-term response rate to nonspecific (placebo) therapies (60% to 80%). The medical management of this disorder has focused on the use of vestibular suppressants (e.g., diazepam, meclizine) to control vertigo, diuretics and a low-salt diet to decrease hydrops, and vasodilators (e.g., niacin, histamine). Of these agents, only vestibular suppressants have been proven to have any beneficial effect in controlling vertigo. No agent has ever been proven to improve auditory function. Nonetheless, many of these agents remain in popular use, with their beneficial effects likely attributable to the nonspecific therapeutic responses seen in this population. Surgical therapies for Meniere's disease involve hearing-preservation approaches (endolymphatic shunt, gentamicin perfusion, vestibular nerve section) or surgeries in which hearing and vestibular function are ablated (labyrinthectomy). Indications for these surgeries are controversial and interested readers are referred to more specialized texts (see immediately below) for an appropriate discussion.

Suggested Readings

Merchant SN, Rauch SD, Nadol JB Jr. Meniere's disease. *Eur Arch Otorhinolaryngol* 252:63–75, 1995.

Ruckenstein MJ, Rutka JA, Hawke M. The treatment of Meniere's disease: Torok revisited. *Laryngoscope* 101:211–218, 1991.

Migrainous Vertigo

The overall course of migrainous vertigo tends to be much more benign than that of Meniere's disease, in that vertiginous episodes tend to be less frequent and the damage to the inner ear tends to be less severe. Vestibular suppressants should be used to suppress the acute vertigo. Although the role of antimigrainous medication in the management of the disorder in these patients has yet to be fully defined, early studies indicate that both prophylactic medications and abortive therapy will likely have a role in the management of this disorder.

Suggested Reading

Bikhazi P, Jackson C, Ruckenstein MJ. Efficacy of antimigrainous therapy in the treatment of migraine-associated dizziness. *Am J Otol* 18:350–354, 1997.

Vestibular Neuronitis

Although the initial episode of vertigo is severe in vestibular neuronitis, symptoms will slowly remit over a period of days to weeks. Vestibular suppressants are the mainstay of treatment of vestibular neuronitis, whereas corticosteroid drugs may well diminish the duration and severity of symptoms if given close to the onset of symptoms. A subgroup of patients will be troubled by persistent imbalance (but not vertigo) subsequent to the resolution of the acute vertigo. This results from a slow compensation of the central nervous system to the altered vestibular input from the damaged peripheral vestibular system. Although most patients will achieve this compensation through normal activities, a small number will need vestibular rehabilitation physical therapy to promote central nervous system compensation to their noncompensated vestibular loss.

Suggested Readings

Ariyasu L, Byl FM, Sprague MS, Adour KK. The beneficial effect of methylprednisolone in acute vestibular vertigo. *Arch Otolaryngol Head Neck Surg* 116:700–703, 1990.

Shepard NT, Telian SA, Smith-Wheelock M, Raj A. Vestibular and balance rehabilitation therapy. *Ann Otol Rhinol Laryngol* 102:198–205, 1993.

Psychogenic Dizziness

Psychogenic dizziness is associated with a variety of psychiatric disorders, most commonly panic, phobic, or chronic anxiety disorders. Although the patient's medical history may be highly suggestive of psychogenic dizziness, a full neuro-otologic history and physical examination must be performed and selective tests are frequently also ordered (e.g., limited MRI, ENG, or dynamic posturography). This is done not only to assure the clinician that no organic disease is present but, perhaps even more important, to reassure the patient.

The treatment of the patient with psychogenic dizziness can be challenging. Often, the patient is convinced that he or she has an organic disease and is reluctant to accept the suggestion that the symptoms may be related to an underlying psychiatric disorder. As with many patients who suffer from somatization disorders, these patients will seek opinions from multiple specialists and will sometimes be given an "organic" diagnosis, such as atypical Meniere's disease. This is indeed unfortunate, as these patients become more convinced that they have organic disease, which further decreases the likelihood that the underlying disorder will be diagnosed. In fact, it is primary care physicians who are best suited to deal with patients with psychogenic dizziness. Because they are most familiar with these patients, they are best able to explore symptoms that may confirm a diagnosis of panic, phobic, or anxiety disorders. Psychiatric referral may be indicated and beneficial. Specific treatments are instituted predicated on the specific psychiatric diagnosis.

Rarer Causes of Vertigo

Three rarer causes of vertigo deserve mention. An acute infection of the inner ear results in vertigo and hearing loss and is termed *labyrinthitis*. Bacterial (suppurative) labyrinthitis results from the spread of meningitis or otitis media to the inner ear and usually results in the complete destruction of the labyrinth. Viral (or serous) labyrinthitis will more commonly result in a partial cochleovestibular loss. Both these entities are considerably rarer then vestibular neuronitis. Suppurative labyrinthitis is treated with drainage of the middle ear (if otitis media is the cause), antibiotics, and corticosteroids, with the prognosis for recovery from this disorder being extremely poor. Serous labyrinthitis is treated with corticosteroids.

An **acoustic neuroma** is a schwannoma of the vestibular nerve that classically presents with asymmetric sensorineural hearing loss. Imbalance, particularly in the dark, is a frequent complaint associated with these slow-growing tumors, with vertigo being a much rarer complaint. Dysfunction of the fifth cranial nerve (hypoesthesia) or—rarely—the seventh cranial nerve (facial paralysis) may also be present. Diagnosis is confirmed with a MRI scan and treatment is typically surgical removal.

For the inner ear to function properly, its fluid compartments must be anatomically separated from surrounding structures. Violation of the barriers between the middle and inner ears can result in symptoms of hearing loss and vertigo known as a **perilymph fistula.** This diagnosis was made frequently during the 1960s and 1970s but is now recognized as being a rare entity. Currently, most otologists would consider the diagnosis if the patient described a history of symptom onset immediately after a physical injury to the ear or a barotrauma (e.g., recent air flight or diving). Positive findings on the fistula test, in which a patient develops symptoms of vertigo and nystagmus during pneumatic otoscopy, is a nonspecific finding that may suggest the presence of fistula. Currently, the only method of confirming this diagnosis is direct observation of the fistula during middle ear exploration. Once identified, the fistula can easily be patched.

Suggested Reading

Rizer FM, House JW. Perilymph fistulas: The House Ear Clinic experience. *Otolaryngol Head Neck Surg* 104:239–243, 1991.

CONCLUSION

The evaluation of the dizzy patient is based primarily on the patient's medical history. If the primary care practitioner routinely incorporates the diagnostic algorithm in this chapter, he or she can be confident that an accurate diagnosis can be derived for the vast majority of patients with the complaint of dizziness, using minimal and selective diagnostic testing.

5

FACIAL PARALYSIS

• Michael J. Ruckenstein, M.D., M.Sc., F.R.C.S.C., F.A.C.S.

Cause and Presentation

A cute-onset facial paralysis can represent an anxiety-provoking and disabling disorder. Fortunately, in the vast majority of cases, an acute facial paralysis represents a self-limited process that carries an excellent prognosis. Nonetheless, not all facial palsies are benign, with the differential diagnosis including infectious, traumatic, neoplastic, ischemic, immunologic, and metabolic causes. The presentation of an acute facial paralysis is variable and highly dependent on the etiology. For example, the paralysis may be unilateral or bilateral, slowly progressive or acute and severe, or associated with signs of systemic or central nervous system (CNS) disease. This chapter describes a practical diagnostic algorithm designed to allow the practitioner to make an accurate diagnosis and institute appropriate therapeutic interventions while making judi cious use of diagnostic tests. The algorithm is based on a ser questions the answers to which will reliably indicate th the paralysis.

Natural History

The natural history of faci pendent on the cause. The m lent prognosis and resolve spc weeks. In general, the various in sis for recovery. Traumatic, idiopa carry a more variable prognosis for ery of facial function resulting fron is poor.

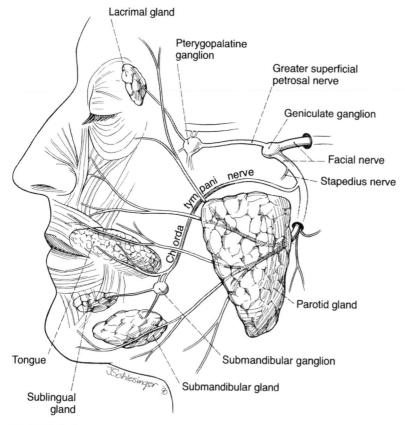

FIGURE 5–1
Course of the facial nerve demonstrating motor branches to the mimetic musculature; parasympathetic innervation to the submandibular, sublingual, lacrimal, and minor salivary glands; and taste fibers emanating from the anterior two thirds of the tongue. (From La Rouere MJ, Kortush JM. Facial nerve paralysis. In Meyerhoff WL, Rice DH [eds.]: *Otolaryngology—Head and Neck Surgery*, Philadelphia: WB Saunders, 1992.)

Diagnosis and Treatment

Are There Symptoms That Point to the Need for Radiologic Workup?

Radiologic workup is indicated when the symptoms suggest the presence of

Neoplasm

tologic pathology

tral nervous system pathology (other than neoplasm; typi-
schemic)

l trauma

ypically involve the facial nerve in the region in
temporal bone (the cerebellopontine angle) or

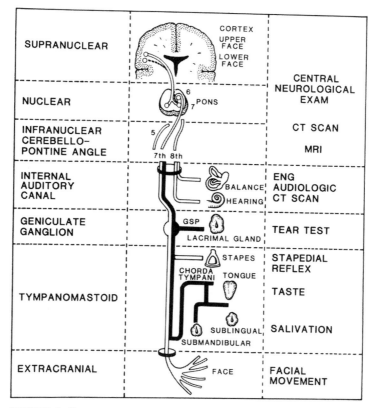

FIGURE 5-2
The anatomy of the facial nerve. (From Shambaugh GE Jr, May M. Facial nerve paralysis. In Paparella MM, Shumrick DA [eds.]: *Otolaryngology*, 2nd ed., Philadelphia: VVB Saunders, 1980.)

within the temporal bone itself. Symptoms suggestive of neoplasm include the following:

- Slow progression of the paralysis over 3 weeks or more

- Recovery that does not begin by 3–6 weeks after onset

- Failure of recovery by 3–6 months

- Facial twitch or spasm preceding the palsy

- History of a previous, ipsilateral palsy (although such a palsy may be associated with Bell's palsy)

- History of multiple cranial nerve deficits (although these may be associated with Bell's palsy)

- Selective sparing of specific motor branches of the facial nerve

Neoplasms involving the facial nerve are typically benign (schwannomas of the seventh or eighth nerve, meningiomas), although metastatic disease or primary CNS malignancies may also be involved. The presence of the above symptoms should prompt the performance of a magnetic resonance imaging (MRI) scan with gadolinium enhancement. Once identified, these lesions will typically require surgical removal.

Mass lesions in the region of the parotid gland can involve the extratemporal component of the facial nerve. These should be readily detectable on physical examination of the neck. The presence of a parotid mass together with a coexistent facial paralysis is highly suggestive of a malignancy and warrants a prompt evaluation by a head and neck surgeon.

Otologic Pathology. Several infectious disorders involving the ear can result in facial paralysis. Thus, an ear examination is absolutely indicated in a patient with facial paralysis.

Malignant Otitis Externa. Necrotizing osteomyelitis of the temporal bone, or malignant otitis externa, is a progressive osteomyelitis of the skull base that spreads from the temporal bone to contiguous structures, involving cranial nerves and ultimately intracranial structures. It is invariably a pseudomonal infection that has classically been reported in patients with diabetes mellitus or other forms of immunocompromise. The hallmark findings are a draining ear with granulations arising off the floor of the ear canal. Confirmation of the diagnosis is made by computed tomography (CT) scan of the temporal bone together with radionuclide scanning. This is an ominous condition that should be managed in consultation with an oto-

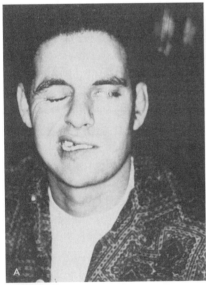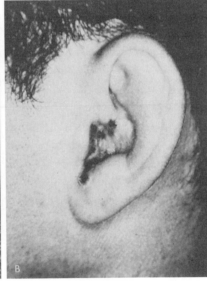

FIGURE 5–3
Herpes zoster oticus. Pain in left ear for 5 days and facial paralysis and herpetic eruption of auricle for 3 days with mild sensorineural high-tone hearing loss and slight dizziness for 2 days. The facial palsy resolved completely in 3 weeks. (Courtesy of Dr. R. I. Barickman; from Shambaugh GE Jr., Glasscock ME III. Facial nerve decompression and repair. In *Surgery of the Ear*, 2nd ed., Philadelphia: WB Saunders, 1980, p 532.)

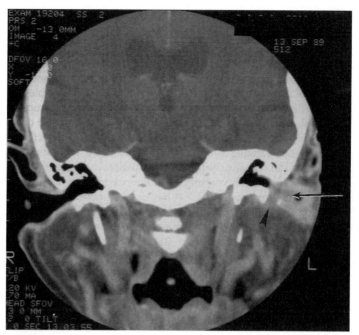

FIGURE 5–4

Necrotizing external otitis with early extension inferiorly. Coronal computed tomography scan shows an area of nonspecific attenuation (*arrow*) in the external auditory canal. Just at the bone–cartilage junction, there is a small area of soft-tissue attenuation (*arrowhead*) extending inferiorly below the limit of the canal (compare with opposite side) that represents early extension through Santorini's fissures. (From Grandis JR, Yu VL. Necrotizing (malignant) external otitis. In Johnson JT, Yu VL [eds.]: *Infectious Diseases and Antimicrobial Therapy of the Ear, Nose, and Throat*, Philadelphia: WB Saunders, 1997.)

laryngologist and a specialist in infectious diseases. Treatment involves prolonged systemic antipseudomonal antibiotics and, in refractory or aggressive disease, surgical debridement.

Acute otitis media can rarely be complicated by facial paralysis. Chronic otitis media (chronic purulent drainage from the ear through a tympanic membrane perforation) can be associated with cholesteatoma formation. A cholesteatoma, which is really an epidermoid cyst arising off the tympanic membrane, can grow medially, resulting in facial paralysis secondary to compression and the secretion of toxins. The development of a facial paralysis in the face of acute or chronic middle ear infection necessitates the performance of a high-resolution CT scan of the temporal bone. In the case of acute otitis media, it can identify coalescent mastoiditis, which would necessitate the performance of a cortical mastoidectomy. In the absence of coalescence of the bony air cells of the mastoid, facial paralysis resulting from acute otitis media is best treated with myringotomy and ventilation tube insertion, together with parenteral antibiotics and corticosteroids. The identification of facial paralysis resulting from cholesteatoma is a surgical emergency, with a CT scan helping to identify the site of involvement of the facial nerve, the extent of the disease, and other structures that may be involved (e.g., brain, inner ear).

Central Nervous System Pathology. A variety of syndromes resulting from CNS ischemia have been described in which facial nerve palsy occurs as part of a constellation of neurologic symptoms. Findings indicating a possible CNS cause for the paralysis include

- Selective loss of volitional or spontaneous facial movements

- Associated weakness of other motor groups

- Multiple cranial nerve deficits (although these are also associated with Bell's palsy)

The presence of findings associated with CNS pathology will typically necessitate the performance of an enhanced MRI scan and the request for input from a neurologist.

Facial paralysis that results from an external blunt or penetrating trauma will require the performance of high-resolution CT scan of the temporal bone to identify the site of lesion and other associated injuries. The management of post-traumatic facial nerve paralysis is controversial and the opinion of a neurosurgeon and an otolaryngologist should be obtained.

Is There Evidence of a Systemic Disease Process?

A host of systemic disease processes have been identified that can cause facial paralysis. In many instances, facial paralysis is a secondary event in relation to the development of the primary manifestations of the illness, thus simplifying the diagnostic process. In cases in which systemic disease is not obvious, a search for occult systemic pathology is certainly not warranted during the initial presentation of an acute unilateral facial paralysis. However, systemic disease is very likely in bilateral simultaneous onset facial paralysis. Thus, a more thorough systemic workup is warranted in these cases.

A variety of infectious agents can lead to the development of facial paralysis. Many of them, such as polio, chickenpox, mumps, syphilis, tetanus, and tuberculosis, manifest classical and well-defined clinical symptomatology. Of particular note are infectious mononucleosis and Lyme disease. Both are associated with bilateral, simultaneous facial paralysis. A patient with facial paralysis and the systemic symptoms associated with these disease processes should undergo appropriate serologic evaluation.

Guillain–Barré syndrome and sarcoidosis are two idiopathic inflammatory syndromes that have been associated with facial paralysis, particularly bilateral simultaneous paralysis. Although the diagnosis of Guillain-Barré syndrome may be evident to the clinician, sarcoidosis may require a more extensive workup before its diagnosis is confirmed.

Melkersson–Rosenthal syndrome is a rare but interesting idiopathic condition characterized by recurrent alternating facial palsy, facial edema, and fissured tongue. Even though it is recurrent, the facial palsy typically resolves. There is no specific treatment for this disorder.

Is There a History of Paralysis Secondary to a Known or Presumed Herpetic Infection?

Ramsay Hunt syndrome is an extremely painful vesicular eruption involving the ear canal and contiguous skin, combined with facial paralysis and sometimes sensorineural hearing loss and vertigo. It is caused by a recrudescence of a herpes zoster infection. Treatment of this disorder should include an antiherpetic agent and corticosteroids.

The reader will note that up until this point, the term *Bell's palsy* has not been used. This was done with the intent of emphasizing that *all facial paralysis is not Bell's.* Rather, the term *Bell's palsy* refers to a disorder primarily characterized by an acute onset of unilateral facial paralysis of variable severity, frequently subsequent to a viral prodrome, with certain associated symptoms. There is frequently (20%–60% of cases) evidence of a sensory cranial nerve polyneuritis including periauricular pain, facial numbness (fifth nerve), hypercusis (sensitivity to sound—eighth nerve), altered taste (seventh and ninth nerves), and numbness of the tongue (ninth nerve). Occasionally, a paralysis of the motor branch of the tenth nerve can be identified. Thus, the presence of an acute facial nerve palsy together with symptoms of a sensory cranial nerve polyneuritis need not provoke an extensive workup as long as symptoms of neoplastic and systemic disease, as described above, are not present.

The treatment of Bell's palsy has long been controversial, owing partly to the high spontaneous recovery rate associated with this disorder. The use of corticosteroids has been debated, but the sum total of clinical evidence is that the administration of corticosteroids early in the course of the paralysis will improve the level of recovery and thus decrease the degree of permanent disability in some patients.

Circumstantial evidence has accumulated supporting the hypothesis that Bell's palsy is caused by the herpes simplex virus. One recent—but somewhat controversial—study has provided some evidence that the early administration of acyclovir may be beneficial in this disorder (see Suggested Readings). The optimal dose and, in fact, even the antiherpetic agent of choice have yet to be established. Nonetheless, many practitioners are treating Bell's palsy with a combination of prednisone and an antiherpetic agent, unless these medications are contraindicated.

Physical Examination

On the basis of the above discussion, it should be apparent that the patient with facial paralysis requires a focused physical examination, including

- Determination of degree and uniformity (i.e., are certain branches spared?) of paralysis

- Otoscopy

- Tuning fork auditory evaluation

- Examination of cranial nerves

- Neck examination (to rule out parotid mass)

Supportive Care in All Types of Facial Paralysis

In addition to specific treatments designed to address the underlying cause of the paralysis, it is critical that the practitioner ensures provision of adequate eye protection to the patient. Patients should be questioned regarding symptoms of exposure keratitis. Suspicion of this disorder should prompt a fluorescein examination of the cornea. All patients with facial paralysis should be given eye protection measures, which include frequent instillation of natural tears during the day, application of Lacrilube ointment at night, and taping the eye shut or application of a moisture chamber, particularly at night. Persistent paralysis should prompt an ophthalmologic evaluation.

Clinicians should also be sympathetic to the fact that persistent facial paralysis can result in significant symptoms of depression in the patient. Counseling, together with antidepressant medication, may be required.

Congenital Facial Nerve Paralysis

When facial paralysis is detected at birth, another differential diagnosis than the one described above for the adult population is applicable. Congenital facial paralysis can be divided into developmental or traumatic categories. Paralysis resulting from developmental disorders is frequently bilateral, incomplete, and associated with other anomalies. Möbius' syndrome is a rare congenital condition characterized by bilateral facial palsy, together with abducens palsy and deformities of the extremities. Myotonic dystrophy is a progressive familial disorder consisting of weakness and wasting of the muscles of the head and neck. Congenital unilateral lower lip paralysis (asymmetric crying facies syndrome) is significant, as it is frequently associated with other anomalies.

By contrast, facial paralysis resulting from birth trauma is typically complete and unilateral. There is frequently evidence of trauma, such as bruising of the head or hematotympanum. Paralysis results from pressure applied to the extratemporal facial nerve by the maternal sacrum, or, less frequently, by obstetrical forceps. The prognosis for the spontaneous recovery from traumatic congenital paralysis is excellent, with most infants showing recovery by 5 weeks of age.

In summary, facial nerve paralysis can most often be diagnosed by clinical evaluation without the need for expensive investigations. Nonetheless, not all facial paralysis is Bell's palsy, so care must be taken to identify those critical findings on medical history and physical examination that point to an alternate diagnosis. Once identified, these findings will lead to a specific and directed evaluation.

When to Refer

Any patient with facial paralysis associated with otologic pathology should be referred to an otolaryngologist for management of the condition. Neoplasms require patient referral to a specialist; the area of expertise chosen depends on the neoplasm's site of origin. Neurologists should be involved in the care of patients with evidence of ischemic, infectious, or idiopathic disease involving the CNS.

Suggested Readings

Adour KK, Byl FM, Hilsinger RL Jr, et al. The true nature of Bell's palsy: analysis of 1,000 consecutive patients. *Laryngoscope* 88:787–801, 1978.

Adour KK, Ruboyianes JM, Von Doersten PG, et al. Bell's palsy treatment with acyclovir and prednisone compared with prednisone alone: A double-blind, randomized, controlled trial. *Ann Otol Rhinol Laryngol* 105:371–378, 1996.

Harris JP, Davidson TM, May M, Fria T. Evaluation and treatment of congenital facial paralysis. *Arch Otolaryngol* 109:145–151, 1983.

May M, Klein SR, Taylor FH. Idiopathic (Bell's) facial palsy: Natural history defies steroid or surgical treatment. *Laryngoscope* 95:406–409, 1985.

6

THE NOSE AND SINUS DISEASE

INTRODUCTION

Nasal congestion and rhinorrhea are extremely common complaints. Allergic rhinitis afflicts 10%–12% of the U.S. population. Sinusitis was the fifth leading cause for antibiotic prescriptions during ambulatory care visits between 1985 and 1992. A 1993 survey reported a 15% incidence of sinusitis that lasted at least 3 months. Rhinosinusitis, although common, is not a trivial illness. Its economic impact is substantial. Between 1990 and 1992, sinusitis accounted for approximately 73 million restricted activity days per year. Quality of life is also significantly affected. The Medical Outcomes Study short-form 36-item survey (SF-36) indicates that patients with chronic sinusitis experience significant decrements in quality-of-life domains, such as general health and social functioning. Moreover, the severity of these effects is as great as that of effects of diseases frequently regarded as more serious, such a chronic obstructive pulmonary disease, congestive heart failure, and angina pectoris. Finally, sinus infections may result in serious complications, such as orbital or intracranial infections.

Definitions

Rhinosinusitis is the inflammation of the nasal cavity and paranasal sinuses. Although rhinitis and sinusitis are widely considered to be separate problems, one rarely occurs without the other. The nasal and sinus cavities are lined by continuous respiratory epithelium, covered by an unbroken mucus blanket. Computed tomography (CT) scanning in patients with uncomplicated common colds demonstrates simultaneous involvement of the nasal and sinus mucosa.

Rhinitis refers to chronic nonsuppurative inflammation of the nasal mucosa. The most common cause of chronic rhinitis is inhalant allergy. Allergic rhinitis may be seasonal, due to pollen allergy, or perennial, in response to constantly present allergens, such as dust. The cause of nonallergic rhinitis is not known, but it is usually elicited by physical stimuli and therefore is probably some form of vasomotor hypersensitivity.

The term *sinusitis* is generally used to refer to infectious suppurative rhinosinusitis, which may be acute or indolent. The United States Food and Drug Administration defines acute sinusitis as an infection lasting up to 4 weeks and chronic sinusitis as an infection persisting after 3 months. The Rhinosinusitis Task Force of the American Academy of Otolaryngology—Head and Neck Surgery has recommended use of the term *subacute sinusitis* for infections lasting more than 4 weeks but less than 12 weeks. Acute and chronic sinusitis differ greatly in symptoms and histopathology.

Acute sinusitis produces significant local discomfort and is pathologically an exudative process, predominated by neutrophils, with necrosis, hemorrhage, and sometimes ulceration. Chronic sinusitis is characterized by a proliferative process with fibrosis of the lamina propria and infiltration by lymphocytes, plasma cells, and eosinophils. The symptoms of chronic sinusitis are more subtle than those of acute sinusitis, as the inflammatory process is more indolent. Uncommonly, surgery for chronic sinusitis reveals allergic fungal sinusitis, with tenacious mucin, fungal hyphae, Charcot–Leyden crystals, and a dense eosinophilic infiltrate. Recurrent acute sinusitis is defined as more than four discrete episodes of sinusitis per year. Recurrent episodes of sinusitis may also occur as acute exacerbations of chronic sinusitis.

Nasal septal deformity is extremely common. Mild to moderate deformity is usually asymptomatic, but more severe deformity can obstruct the nasal passages, predispose the patient to sinus infections, or be implicated in headaches. Nasal septal deformity consists of deviation of the nasal septum and/or spurs projecting into the nasal cavity. Such deformity may result from trauma or from normal anatomic variation. Mild septal deformity is extremely common and usually has no clinical significance. Moderate to severe nasal septal deformity can cause nasal obstruction or increased susceptibility to sinus infection.

Chronic Rhinitis

Presentation and Progression

Chronic inflammation of the nasal mucosa produces the clinical symptoms of sneezing, nasal congestion, and rhinorrhea. In most patients, these symptoms are due to inhalant allergy. Cell-bound immunoglobulin E in the nasal mucosa reacts with specific antigens, causing the release of chemical mediators. In the early phase, mast cells release such substances as histamine, prostaglandin, and kinins. In the late-phase reaction, other inflammatory cells, such as eosinophils and basophils, secrete further mediators. Even a brief exposure to an allergen can result in symptoms that last for days. Patients with seasonal rhinitis are usually sensitive to pollens. Symptoms are maximal in spring and/or autumn, correlating with atmospheric levels of pollen. Patients with perennial allergic rhinitis are usually sensitive to ubiquitous household allergens, such as dust, mold, and mites.

A second major form of chronic nasal complaints is nonallergic rhinitis also known as vasomotor rhinitis. This appears to be an autonomic rather than immunologic problem with hypersensitivity to physical stimuli, such as temperature changes, pollution, fumes, and tobacco smoke. A third form, "rhinitis medicamentosa," results from habitual use of topical decongestant nasal sprays.

Diagnosis

The cause of chronic nasal symptoms can usually be discerned from findings on the medical history and physical. However, this task is complicated by the fact that various disease processes result in similar signs and symptoms. Both allergic and infectious processes are associated with nasal congestion, thick secretions, fatigue, and persistent cough. A diagnosis of allergic rhinitis is supported by the complaints of itching of the eyes and nose, clear rhinorrhea, and frequent sneezing. Seasonal variation also favors an allergic cause, as does a history that links the symptoms to specific situations or allergen exposures, such as dust, smoke, fumes, or certain strong odors.

Nasal obstruction may be continuous or intermittent or may occur only when the patient is recumbent. It may be unilateral or bilateral, or both sides may be variably affected. Unilateral obstruction suggests an anatomic cause, such as nasal septal deviation or turbinate hypertrophy, obstruction by polyps, or even a tumor. Variable obstruction suggests an inflammatory cause. Both anatomic and inflammatory obstructions are worse when the patient is recumbent and may become manifest only when the patient retires for the night.

The quality of nasal discharge may suggest the cause. Profuse, watery rhinorrhea is most suggestive of allergy, but an abundance of eosinophil exudate can occur, rendering nasal secretions cloudy. Colored or malodorous discharge indicates infection. Does the nose spontaneously run, or is discharge noted on blowing the nose or clearing secretions from the throat? Profuse watery discharge that varies with position or exertion may indicate a cerebrospinal fluid leak!

A complaint of postnasal drip does not necessarily indicate nasal discharge. Mucus glands in the nose and sinuses produce approximately 1 L of mucus per day under normal conditions. This mucus is continuously propelled by cilia out of the sinuses, through the nasal cavity, and into the pharynx, where it is swallowed. In most cases, a perception of postnasal drip reflects not an increase in the quantity of nasal secretions but either a change in the viscosity of the mucus or inflammation and swelling in the pharynx. Efforts to clear the throat can exacerbate this problem.

A medication history is very important in evaluating patients with nasal complaints. Nasal obstructions are a side effect of many drugs, including reserpine, hydralazine, propranolol, methyldopa, thioridazine, chlordiazepoxide, amitriptyline, perphenazine, and contraceptives. A history of aspirin sensitivity may be elicited in patients with asthma and nasal polyps. Additionally, the vast majority of patients with chronic rhinitis have taken medications—over-the-counter preparations and/or prescriptions—for their problems in the past. Response to prior medication can help to identify the cause of the problem.

A favorable response to antihistamine therapy, with decreased secretions and itching, is strong support for an allergic cause. However, many preparations include a sympathomimetic decongestant in addition to an antihistamine; therefore, it is important to establish the precise preparation taken. A response to decongestant therapy is not useful diagnostically, as mucosal vasoconstriction can improve nasal patency even in patients with fixed anatomic obstruction. Improvement with antibiotic therapy implicates infection.

Patients who report frequent use of topical nasal decongestant spray probably have developed "rhinitis medicamentosa." The vasoconstriction induced by the nasal spray can actually result in relative ischemia, and reperfusion results in hyperemia and edema. In an effort to maintain nasal patency, patients increase the frequency of decongestant use. The result is not just an "addiction" to topical nasal spray but also a pathologic change in the nasal mucosa. "Rhinitis medicamentosa" usually occurs in patients with other rhinologic pathology, but optimal management of the underlying pathology requires that the nasal spray problem be resolved first. In particular, surgery should be deferred until well after the nasal decongestant spray has been discontinued. This is because local hyperemia and decreased vascular contractility result in increased bleeding, both during and after surgery.

Nonallergic rhinitis is chiefly a diagnosis of exclusion. Symptoms are quite similar to those of perennial allergic rhinitis or chronic sinusitis. However, antihistamines offer little or no benefit. One helpful piece of information from the history is that patients with nonallergic rhinitis quite often note provocation or exacerbation of their symptoms by physical stimuli, such as changes in temperature or humidity.

Physical examination in a patient with rhinitis of any cause reveals variable degrees of turbinate congestion and rhinorrhea. The mucosa in noninfectious rhinitis is pale and may have a bluish cast. Chronic inflammation may cause "cobblestoning" of the mucosa. Application of a topical decongestant spray improves visualization of the nasal cavity for evaluation of the septum and identification of nasal polyps or tumors. Septal deformities are extremely common. Mild abnormalities generally do not impair nasal breathing under normal conditions but may reduce the tolerance for swelling caused by rhinitis. Septal perforation is unusual and suggests prior surgery, autoimmune disorder, or cocaine abuse.

Nasal polyps arise from the upper lateral walls of the nasal cavity, between the turbinates. Nasal polyps can occur in patients with allergy, but polyps are not a pathognomonic physical sign of allergy. More often, polyps are associated with nonallergic asthma.

Plain x-rays are not often useful in managing chronic rhinitis. If sinus infection is suspected, a Water's projection radiograph may confirm the diagnosis by demonstrating fluid in the maxillary sinus. False negatives are quite common, as sinusitis is frequently localized to the ethmoid sinuses, which are poorly visualized with plain films. Computed tomography (CT) scanning is the most accurate means of imaging the sinuses; however, its expense cannot be justified in the majority of cases.

Nasal cytology has been recommended as a simple office-based test to determine the cause of chronic nasal symptoms. Studies from many years ago indicated that allergy, bacterial infection, viral infection, and vasomotor rhinitis each produced different types of inflammatory cells in nasal secretions. Eosinophils were thought to indicate allergy, whereas neutrophils were predominant in the presence of infection. However, no recent investigators have confirmed the validity of nasal cytology. Eosinophils may be abundant in the secretions of patients with nonallergic rhinitis. Moreover, many patients with rhinitis are already being treated with topical nasal steroids, which can decrease the number of eosinophils. Thus, nasal cytology is not currently considered to be a useful test.

SUMMARY OF DIAGNOSIS

Allergic Rhinitis

- Sneezing, congestion, clear rhinorrhea, and/or itching eyes
- Seasonal (spring and/or fall) or perennial
- Beneficial response to antihistamines
- Radiographs and laboratory tests generally not needed

Vasomotor Rhinitis

- Sneezing, congestion, and/or clear rhinorrhea
- Symptoms provoked by temperature and humidity changes
- No benefit from an antihistamine
- Radiographs and laboratory tests generally not needed

Natural History

The onset of symptoms of nasal allergy is usually during childhood or adolescence. Severity usually increases over the next two to three years, and then stabilizes. Symptoms usually diminish in old age. Approximately one fifth of patients with allergic rhinitis also have asthma, but the two problems do not necessarily become manifest at the same time. The symptoms of allergic rhinitis are generally annoying rather than incapacitating. However, rhinitis can lead to infectious complications, such as sinusitis and otitis media. It has also been suggested that chronic mouth breathing in rhinitis patients may predispose to tonsil infections.

Treatment

Allergic rhinitis can usually be managed symptomatically with medications, including oral antihistamines and decongestants and topical steroid or cromolyn spray. Antihistamines are useful to decrease the frequency and severity of reactions to allergens. The newer nonsedating antihistamines are preferable. The older antihistamine preparations cause not only drowsiness but also thickening of secretions. Altered secretions can impair mucus clearance, which may result in sinus infection. Systemic decongestants, such as pseudoephedrine, provide nonspecific reduction of nasal congestion. Intranasal steroid sprays are highly effective in reducing edema and inflammation but require about 2 weeks to achieve maximal effect. Thus, it is prudent to use an oral medication initially, tapering off as tolerated when the effects of the spray appear. Nasal steroids can safely be used in the long term in patients with perennial rhinitis, or intermittently in patients with seasonal rhinitis. Topical cromolyn spray is also beneficial in allergic rhinitis but requires frequent application. In patients with profuse, watery discharge, topical ipratropium bromide can be helpful in diminishing secretions.

Treatment of nonallergic rhinitis is similar to treatment of allergic rhinitis, including systemic decongestants and cromolyn or steroid sprays. Antihistamines are ineffective.

When to Refer

When medical therapy is inadequate to control symptoms, allergy testing is indicated. Skin testing or radioallergosorbent testing can be used to identify specific allergens. Patients can then be instructed to avoid specific allergens or may undergo desensitization. Physicians who use skin testing or administer desensitization must be trained and must have offices equipped to manage anaphylaxis. Allergy testing may also reveal that the patient has a nonallergic form of rhinitis.

If medical therapy or desensitization is inadequate, surgical options can address specific problems. In patients with recalcitrant nasal congestion, surgical resection can reduce the size of the inferior turbinates. Alternatively, engorgement of turbinates can be diminished by coagulation of submucosal vessels using electrocautery, laser, or cryotherapy. Correction of any septal deformity may also be beneficial. Surgical resection can be used to reduce the size of the inferior turbinates.

KEY POINTS

— Diagnosis is primarily based on findings on the medical history and physical examination.

— The symptom of postnasal drip does not reflect nose or sinus disease.

— Allergic rhinitis may be seasonal or perennial.

— Medical management can control most symptoms.

— Allergy testing is indicated when medical management fails.

— Desensitization to specific antigens often provides relief.

— Surgery may be of benefit in selected patients.

Suggested Readings

Mabry RL. Pharmacotherapy with immunotherapy for the treatment of otolaryngic allergy. *Ear Nose Throat J* 69:63–71, 1990.

Mygand N, Naclerio RM. *Allergic and Non-Allergic Rhinitis: Clinical Aspects.* Copenhagen: Munksgaard; Philadelphia: WB Saunders, 1993.

Nasal Septal Deformity

Slight irregularities of the bone and cartilage making up the nasal septum are frequently observed, and in fact, a perfectly straight septum is uncommon. Deviations of the septum and spurs projecting into the nasal cavity occur as a result of anatomic variation or of trauma. Some types of septal nasal deformity seem to run in families and many others are probably the result of birth trauma. Most patients with severe nasal deformity have a history of prior nasal trauma. Fracture of the nasal septum usually accompanies fracture of the nasal bones but may occur in isolation. Septal deviation and spurs often present long after the original trauma, as the septal injury becomes exaggerated over time.

The most common clinical presentation of nasal septal deformity is chronic nasal obstruction. Nasal obstruction is worse at night and may result in sleep disturbances. Septal deformity may also present as frequent sinus infections. Spurs and deviation of the nasal septum may also result in recurrent nosebleeds.

Diagnosis

Nasal septal deformity is apparent on physical inspection of the nose. In some cases, the septum "bulges" to one side in the center. In other patients, there is an S-shaped deviation that occludes both nasal cavities. An old fracture line can frequently be appreciated. Bone spurs may project into the nasal cavity.

Nasal septal deformity is also well demonstrated by CT scanning. In fact, some insurance companies now require CT documentation of septal deviation before authorizing surgical treatment. However, CT is quite expensive and its cost is difficult to justify.

Natural History

Nasal septal deformity does not often present before adolescence, even when caused by a fracture sustained in birth or childhood. Deviations and spurs, whether due to trauma or to anatomic variation, usually begin to develop during the nasal growth spurt but may not be clinically obvious until several years later. Septal deformity due to a fracture sustained in adulthood is usually immediately apparent but may also develop as a delayed complication.

Treatment

Most patients with mild to moderate nasal obstruction have no clinical signs or symptoms. In other patients, medical control of nasal allergies results in a satisfactory airway. However, definitive treatment of nasal septal deformity is surgical correction.

When to Refer

Significant nasal obstruction, recurrent sinus infections, and recurrent epistaxis are all valid indications for surgical correction of nasal septal deformity.

Nasal Polyposis

Nasal polyps are benign inflammatory masses that arise from sinus mucosa and project into the nasal cavity. The cause of nasal polyps is unknown. They occur frequently in patients with asthma and sometimes as part of a triad of nasal polyps, asthma, and aspirin sensitivity. Nasal polyposis in children is highly suggestive of cystic fibrosis. Clinically, polyps present as nasal obstruction and sometimes as loss of smell. Polyps can also cause recurrent sinus infections and occasionally expansion of the nasal dorsum.

Diagnosis

Nasal polyps are detected on physical examination. They first become apparent superiorly, but when they are advanced, they can fill the entire nasal cavity. They usually have a characteristic bluish, glossy, translucent appearance.

Treatment

There is no known cure for nasal polyposis. Polyps nearly always recur after surgical excision, even when this includes radical opening of sinuses. Systemic and topical steroids can retard growth, sometimes delaying or eliminating the need for repeat surgery.

When to Refer

Otolaryngology consultation is indicated in any patient suspected of having nasal polyposis. Biopsy is required to establish the diagnosis and rule out nasal tumor. Treatment is control of polyp growth by systemic and topical steroids and surgical excision as needed.

Other Conditions Presenting with Nasal Obstruction

Nasal obstruction and epistaxis in a male adolescent suggest possible nasopharyngeal angiofibroma. This is an extremely vascular and benign but locally invasive tumor. Physical examination demonstrates a mass lesion in the nasopharynx or posterior nasal cavity. Diagnosis is established by CT with contrast. Biopsy is not recommended, as it is likely to result in severe hemorrhage. Treatment is by surgical excision, if resectable. When there is intracranial spread, radiotherapy—and sometimes chemotherapy—is indicated.

Acute Sinusitis

A fundamental mechanism involved in nearly all cases of bacterial rhinosinusitis is impairment of mucus clearance. Normal nasal and sinus mucosa generates approximately 1 L of mucus each day. This is normally propelled from the sinuses by cilia through the posterior choana to the pharynx, where it is swallowed. If clearance is impaired for any reason, then secretions pool in the sinuses, serving as fertile culture media for bacteria. Clearance may be impaired by mechanical obstruction, increased viscosity of mucus, or decreased ciliary function.

Acute bacterial rhinosinusitis most commonly occurs as a complication of a viral upper respiratory infection (URI). Mucosal swelling can occlude sinus ostia, and the viral infection can also directly impair ciliary function. Other causes of mucosal inflammation, such as allergy and gastroesophageal reflux, can result in sinusitis. Nasal passages and ostia may be smaller than normal on the basis of anatomic variation, with a decreased tolerance for swelling, and consequently an increased susceptibility to sinus infections. Other anatomic variations associated with an increased incidence of sinusitis include nasal septum deviation and turbinate malformations, such as concha bullosa or paradoxical middle turbinate (Fig. 6–1).

Presentation

Abrupt onset of nasal congestion and rhinorrhea with a duration of a few days most likely represents a viral URI or an acute allergic event. When acute symptoms (Table 6–1) do not resolve within 1 week or become worse after 4 or 5 days, the patient is presumed to have a bacterial infection.

Diagnosis

The medical history and physical examination findings are generally sufficient to establish the diagnosis of acute infectious rhinosinusitis.

A   B

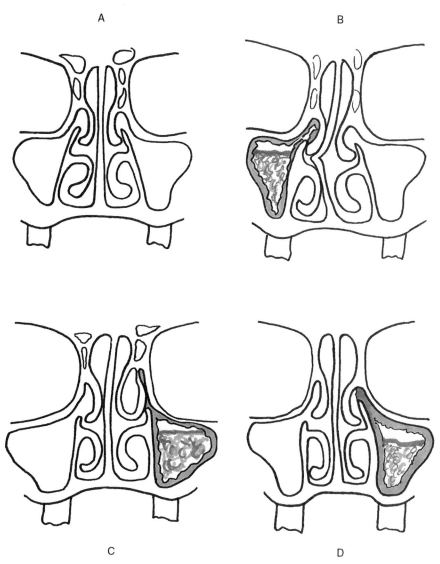

C   D

FIGURE 6–1

Anatomic variations which increase the incidence of sinus infections (coronal sections midway through nose, including middle and inferior turbinates, maxillary sinuses, and portions of ethmoids): **A,** normal; **B,** deviation of nasal septum, occluding middle meatus; **C,** concha bullosa (air cell in middle turbinate); **D,** tall uncinate process, blocking maxillary outflow.

The most common symptoms are headache, nasal congestion, and thick nasal discharge.

Common signs of acute sinusitis are nasal obstruction or congestion, purulent nasal discharge, facial pressure or pain, decreased smell, dental pain, sore throat, otitis, cough, and fever.

Intranasal examination usually reveals hyperemic and swollen nasal mucosa. Topical decongestion is required for adequate inspection. However, this should be applied after initial perusal, to permit assessment of unaltered mucosal color and congestion. Decongestion

TABLE 6–1 • **COMMON SIGNS OF ACUTE SINUSITIS**

Nasal obstruction or congestion
Purulent nasal discharge
Facial pressure or pain
Decreased smell
Dental pain
Sore throat
Otitis
Cough
Fever

should of course be approached judiciously in patients with cardiac disease or hypertension. For this reason, Neo-Synephrine is generally the preferred agent.

Palpation of the face can elicit important diagnostic cues. Tenderness over the cheek or upper gum indicates acute maxillary inflammation. Ethmoid sinusitis results in tenderness of the lacrimal area. Frontal sinus tenderness is maximal over the sinus floor, under the medial portion of the superior orbital rim. However, tenderness is frequently not present; therefore, absence of facial tenderness does not rule out an acute sinus infection.

A careful evaluation of cranial nerve function, including visual acuity, is essential to monitor for potential orbital or intracranial complications. Abducens weakness or pupillary sluggishness is an ominous sign of possible cavernous sinus involvement. Mental status changes or altered consciousness are other red flags.

Plain Sinus X-rays. In the management of rhinosinusitis, plain sinus x-rays are of limited value. Maxillary sinusitis is usually quite apparent on a Water's projection (Fig. 6–2). However, the ethmoid sinuses, which are most frequently involved in sinusitis, are not adequately demonstrated by plain radiographs. Thus, false negatives are extremely common.

Computed Tomography. The imaging technique of choice in the evaluation of sinusitis is CT. It images all sinuses, demonstrating sinus opacification, mucosal thickening, and bony anatomy (Fig. 6–3). Computed tomography scanning is expensive and time consuming and is not necessary for the initial diagnosis and management of incipient acute sinusitis. However, it is essential when orbital or intracranial complications are suspected. In such cases, scans should be performed with and without intravenous contrast, and the intracranial cavity should be included in the scan.

Ultrasound. Ultrasound is not particularly helpful in the management of sinusitis because it can be used to evaluate only the maxillary sinuses. If a sinus is filled with air, virtually all the sound

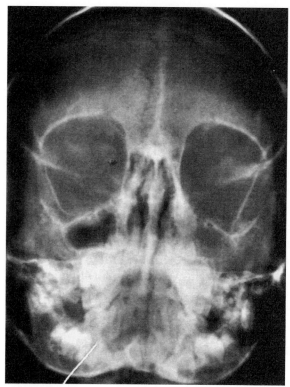

FIGURE 6-2
Water's projection sinus radiograph showing maxillary sinus opacification. (From Wald ER. Rhinitis and acute and chronic sinusitis. In Bluestone CD, Stool SE, Kenna MA. [eds.]: *Pediatric Otolaryngology*, 3rd ed., Philadelphia: WB Saunders, 1996.)

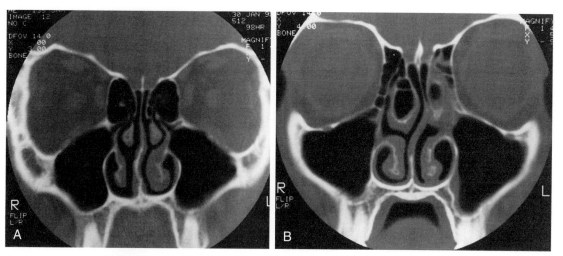

FIGURE 6-3
Coronal computed tomography scan of sinuses: **A,** normal findings; **B,** concha bullosa and ethmoid sinusitis.

is reflected by the anterior edge of the air space. However, if the sinus is filled with pus, sound waves will travel through the sinus and be reflected by the posterior wall. Ultrasound is more sensitive and less specific than plain x-rays and is far inferior to CT. Ultrasound has a sensitivity of 58% and a specificity of 55%. Both air between the anterior sinus wall and pus in the sinus will result in a false negative.

Transillumination. An old technique that is easy to use, transillumination does not require sophisticated equipment. It does require a dark room and a specially covered lightbulb. For evaluation of the frontal sinus, the light is covered by a sheath (which transmits light only through a flat plate at the end). The light tip is placed against the medial orbital roof, just posterior to the orbital rim (Fig. 6–4). The light should be flush against the skin so that no light leaks directly into the room. The ipsilateral frontal sinus should appear as a reddish glow above the eyebrow. For evaluation of the maxillary

CRITERIA FOR DIAGNOSIS OF ACUTE SINUSITIS

Temporal Criteria

Acute: ≤ 4 weeks' duration
Subacute: 4–12 weeks' duration
Recurrent acute: ≥ 4 episodes per year, each lasting ≥ 7 days, with no intervening symptoms

Clinical Factors

Major:
    Facial pain/pressure
    Facial congestion/fullness
    Nasal obstruction/blockage
    Nasal discharge/purulence/discolored postnasal discharge
    Decreased or absent smell

Minor:
    Headache
    Halitosis
    Fatigue
    Dental pain
    Cough
    Ear pressure/fullness

Diagnostic Certainty

Strong:
    ≥ 2 major factors
        or
    1 major + 2 minor factors
        or
    Nasal purulence on examination
Suggestive:
    1 major factor
        or
    ≥ 2 minor factors

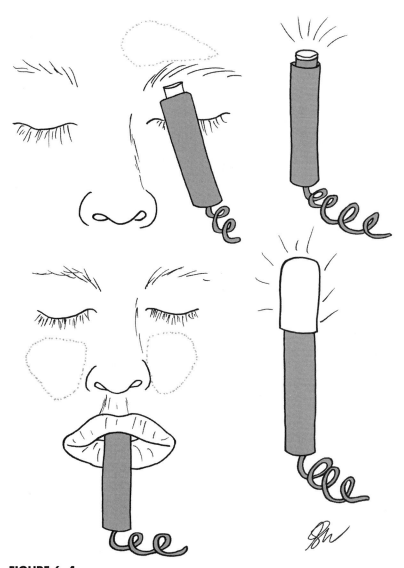

FIGURE 6-4
Technique of sinus transillumination. Dotted lines indicate transilluminated areas. Light sources shown at right. *Upper panel,* frontal sinus; *lower panel,* maxillary sinus.

sinuses, the light sheath should transmit circumferentially. The light is placed into the patient's mouth. The patient is instructed to seal the lips around the light but to leave the jaws open. Both maxillary sinuses should appear in the malar areas. Transillumination can be a useful adjunct in following some cases, demonstrating resolution of maxillary fluid. It is fun to perform and offers virtually no risk to the patient. However, its findings should not be the sole basis for a treatment decision, as its sensitivity and specificity are far inferior to that of CT.

Cultures are usually not helpful in the management of acute sinusitis. Specimens obtained by intranasal swabs are poor indicators of sinus pathogens. Moreover, the commonly encountered organisms are well known, so that empiric therapy is indicated.

Natural History

Acute sinusitis is most often a self-limited disease, even without antibiotic therapy, but many patients develop chronic or recurrent infections. Antibiotic therapy hastens resolution of symptoms of acute sinusitis. However, antibiotic therapy does not necessarily prevent progression to chronic sinusitis, particularly if antibiotics are discontinued as soon as symptoms resolve. Asymptomatic patients may harbor residual infected mucus in the sinus cavities. This occult infection may smolder and eventually result in a flare-up of recurrent acute infection.

Sinusitis can occasionally lead to severe complications, including orbital infections, intracranial abscesses, meningitis, and cavernous sinus thrombosis. The predominant spread of infection in such cases is usually not directly through bone but through the venous drainage system. In this danger zone, veins draining the sinuses, midface, and intracranial cavity are interconnected and lack valves. It is important to be vigilant for signs of possible intracranial complications. High fever, severe headache, neck pain, drowsiness, and visual disturbances are red flags that should be investigated.

Orbital complications of sinusitis are most commonly encountered in children and are often the presenting sign of a latent sinus infection. Eyelid edema and erythema, chemosis, proptosis, and visual disturbance are all signs of orbital infection. Computed tomography is required to differentiate cellulitis from subperiosteal or orbital abscess and to look for potential intracranial complications.

Treatment

Antibiotics are usually indicated in patients diagnosed with acute sinusitis. Most infections are due to *Streptococcus pneumoniae* or *Haemophilus influenzae* (Table 6–2). Amoxicillin is a reasonable choice as a first-line agent. Other options include clarithromycin, cefprozil, loracarbef, and cefaclor, and trimethoprim/sulfamethoxazole. Second-line choices, for recurrent or persistent infection, include amoxicillin–clavulanate, third-generation cephalosporins, levofloxacin, and clindamycin. Antibiotics that are not recommended include penicillin, erythromycin, cephalexin, and tetracycline.

Antibiotic therapy should be continued for several days after symptoms subside, usually for a total of 10 days to 2 weeks. A short course of antibiotics can relieve symptoms but leave a smoldering latent infection or residual contaminated mucus, so that symptomatic infection reemerges a week or more later. There is one possible excep-

TABLE 6–2 • **COMMON CAUSES OF ACUTE SINUSITUS**

Agent	Percent of Cases
Streptococcus pneumoniae	20–41
Haemophilus influenzae	6–50
S. pneumoniae and H. influenzae	1–9
Moraxella (Branhamella) catarrhalis	2–4
S. pyogenes	1–8
Other streptococcal species	2
Staphylococcus aureus	0–8

(From Gwaltney JM. Management of acute sinusitis in adults. In Johnson TT, Yu VL [eds.]: *Infectious Diseases and Antimicrobial Therapy of the Ear, Nose and Throat,* Philadelphia: WB Saunders, 1997, p 344.)

tion to these guidelines for treatment duration. Zithromax is reported to be effective with only 5 days of administration.

Systemic decongestants and short-term use of topical decongestants can alleviate nasal obstruction in patients with acute sinusitis. Topical decongestants should be used sparingly because of the potential for rebound congestion and even "addiction." However, they can provide significant symptomatic relief, particularly at night, when recumbency increases congestion. Decongestion is also probably effective in improving sinus drainage by increasing the patency of the maxillary sinus ostium and the nasal cavity. No studies have been conducted to determine the outcomes benefit of decongestants. Nevertheless, widespread clinical observation through the years has indicated efficacy. In particular, topical decongestion in the clinic can rapidly and dramatically facilitate drainage and hasten symptomatic improvement. Topical decongestants should generally not be used for more than 3 days. A long-acting preparation, such as oxymetazoline, is recommended, because it can be used at bedtime to provide relief throughout the night.

Humidification is frequently advocated in the management of sinusitis, but there is no real data to support its benefit. Moreover, humidifiers tend to grow mold, which can stimulate an allergic response. Mucolytic agents (guaifenesin preparations) have documented benefits in the management of sinusitis.

Antihistamines are usually not helpful in the management of sinusitis. Many antihistamines may even contribute to persistence of the infection because they cause secretions to become thicker and more tenacious. If antihistamines are used to treat concomitant allergic rhinitis, then one of the newer nonsedating drugs should be used, because these have less impact on secretions. Antihistamines are most useful after the acute infection, to prevent or treat acute allergic flares, thereby reducing the chances of recurrent infection.

Ipratropium bromide should be avoided during acute sinusitis because it could lead to stasis of secretions, thereby prolonging the infection or predisposing to recurrence.

The severity of symptoms of acute sinusitis should lessen within 3–4 days after initiation of antibiotic therapy. If symptoms persist or worsen, the choice of antibiotic should be carefully reviewed. Systemic steroids may be helpful to reduce swelling and promote drainage. Computed tomography scanning may be indicated to detect potential complications and to confirm that the pathologic process is indeed a sinus infection. In some cases, sinus irrigation or even acute surgical drainage of the sinuses may be necessary to control the infection.

When to Refer

Otolaryngologic consultation should be considered in patients with acute sinusitis whose condition does not respond as expected to medical therapy. When symptoms of maxillary or upper tooth pain predominate, maxillary sinus irrigation may be indicated in some cases, a measure that can be both therapeutic and diagnostic. Prior to the availability of antibiotics, this was an important therapeutic tool for treating sinus infections. Sinus irrigations are performed much less frequently in recent years, probably because of improved pharmacotherapy.

In adults and cooperative older children, maxillary sinus irrigation can be performed easily in the clinic under local anesthesia (Fig. 6–5). Although it is a simple procedure, it requires hands-on training. The most common approach is via the nose, through the inferior meatus, using a needle or trocar. An alternate approach is to puncture the anterior sinus wall under the upper lip (avoiding the canine tooth root). The patient should then lean forward over a large container, which can catch the fluid that will drain from the nose, and sometimes the mouth. Warmed sterile saline is used to irrigate the cavity; avoid using excessive pressure. The usual result is cloudy fluid, but frequently a large mass of inspissated mucus can be expressed. Irrigation should continue until only clear fluid is obtained. As a final step, negative pressure should be applied to the needle or trocar to aspirate residual fluid and *pull* air into the sinuses. Air should not be *injected* into the sinus, as this could result in potentially fatal air embolism. Misplacement of the cannula can result in injection of fluid into spaces other than the sinus, such as the orbit.

Acute frontal sinusitis may also require irrigation, but this is a surgical procedure that must be accomplished in the operating room. A frontal sinus trephination involves drilling a hole in the floor of the frontal sinus via a small skin incision (Fig. 6–6). A tube is usually left in the sinus for several days for intermittent irrigation, until sterile saline injected into the sinus is noted to drain into the nose. More recently, persisting or severe sinusitis has been approached endoscopically, to reestablish drainage via normal routes.

Acute surgical drainage of the sinuses is definitely indicated in patients with life-threatening complications, such as cavernous sinus

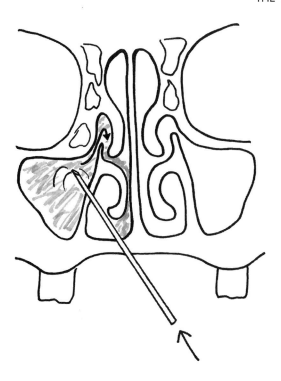

FIGURE 6–5
Technique of maxillary sinus irrigation.

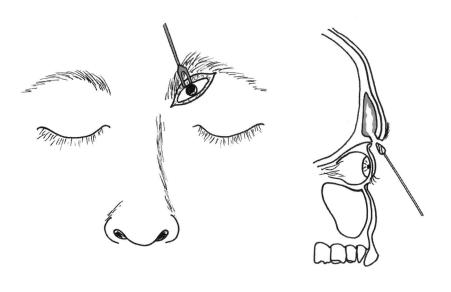

A   B

FIGURE 6–6
Technique of frontal sinus trephination: **A,** anterior view; **B,** sagittal section.

thrombosis, intracranial abscess, or infection. It is also necessary in most patients with orbital infections.

KEY POINTS

— Acute sinusitis most often occurs as a complication of the common cold.

— Purulent rhinorrhea lasting more than 1 week should be treated with antibiotics.

— High fever, headache, and orbital symptoms are warning signs of potential complications.

Suggested Readings

Gwaltney JM. Management of acute sinusitis in adults. In: Johnson JT, Yu VL (eds.): *Infectious Diseases and Antimicrobial Therapy of the Ears, Nose, and Throat.* Philadelphia: WB Saunders, 1997, pp 341–349.

Gwaltney JM, Phillips CD, Miller RD, et al. Computed tomographic study of the common cold. *N Engl J Med* 330:25–30, 1994.

Hamory BH, Sande MA, Snydor A Jr, et al. Etiology and antimicrobial therapy of acute maxillary sinusitis. *J Infect Dis* 139:197–202, 1979.

Chronic Sinusitis

Chronic sinusitis is frequently manifested only by its secondary effects, such as cough or exacerbation of asthma. Sore throat, halitosis, hoarseness, and postnasal drip are also common presentations of chronic sinusitis. Ear symptoms, due to inflammation of the eustachian tube, may also be the presenting signs of chronic sinus infection. Negative pressure, fluid, or acute suppurative otitis media can produce ear pain or pressure, hearing loss, and dizziness. Epistaxis may also be the presenting sign of chronic sinusitis, particularly in children.

Presentation

The clinical presentation of chronic sinusitis is variable. Signs and symptoms are usually subtle because the inflammatory process is indolent. Contrary to popular belief, headache is not a characteristic sign of uncomplicated chronic sinusitis. The most common presentation (Table 6–3) is nasal obstruction, with or without thick nasal secretions. Chronically infected sinuses are frequently filled with inspissated mucus, with no drainage. Other signs include fatigue, cough, and a sensation of facial fullness.

TABLE 6–3 · **COMMONS SIGNS OF CHRONIC SINUSITIS**

Nasal obstruction or congestion
Purulent nasal discharge
Facial pressure or pain
Cough, exacerbation of asthma
Eustachian tube dysfunction
Decreased sense of smell
Halitosis
Fatigue
Sore throat
Otitis
Headache
Postnasal drip

Diagnosis

In the majority of cases, chronic sinusitis can be diagnosed on the basis of findings on the medical history and physical. Chronic sinusitis should be suspected in patients with chronic nasal congestion. As in any nasal complaint, a medication history is very important for detecting the use of drugs that can cause nasal congestion and for determining how the patient has responded to previous therapeutic attempts. A prior beneficial response to antibiotics, however short-lived, is strong evidence for an infectious process.

The location of facial pain or pressure can help in localizing the infection to a specific paranasal sinus. This is important in patients who may require surgery. Maxillary sinus pain is perceived in the cheek or upper teeth. Frontal sinus pain occurs in the forehead and supraorbital rim. Ethmoid sinus involvement produces periorbital and retro-orbital pain. Sphenoid involvement may also result in peri-orbital and retro-orbital symptoms, but the classic site of pain is the vertex of the skull.

Purulence evident on intranasal examination is a definite indicator of sinus infection but is not required for the diagnosis of chronic sinusitis. Sometimes only crusts, the residue of dried purulence, can be observed. Often no drainage can be detected because the sinus is filled with inspissated material or its ostium is occluded.

Computed Tomography. When the diagnosis is apparent because of findings on the medical history and physical examination, CT is not required. However, in some cases, it plays an important role in diagnosis and management. When sinusitis is suspected on the basis of secondary symptoms, such as cough or ear disease, CT scanning can determine whether the sinuses are actually infected (Fig. 6–7). Scanning is also important in the preoperative assessment of patients with infection that is recalcitrant to medical therapy, to determine whether surgery is indicated and to provide a road map for

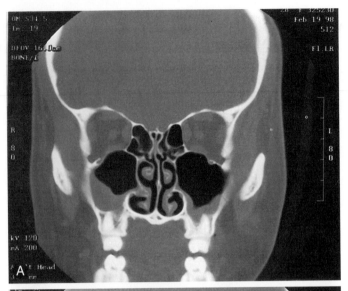

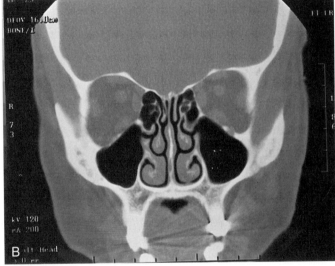

FIGURE 6–7
Computed tomography of sinuses: **A,** bilateral maxillary sinusitis; **B,** enlarged turbinates.

surgery. Computed tomography imaging with intravenous contrast is essential when orbital or intracranial complications are suspected.

Magnetic Resonance Imaging. Magnetic resonance imaging (MRI) offers additional useful information in some cases. It is best for tracking intracranial complications of sinus infection or for evaluating patients with suspected fungal sinusitis (Fig. 6–8). Virtually all acute bacterial and viral infections have bright signal intensities on T_2-weighted images. By contrast, fungal infection has either a low signal or no signal. The major limitation of MRI is that it does not demonstrate bone, so it cannot be used to plan surgery.

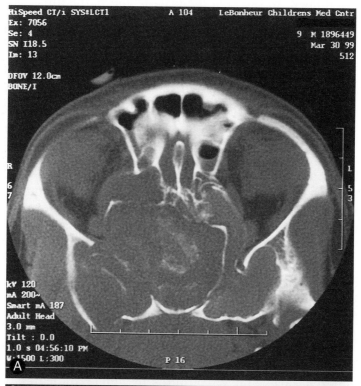

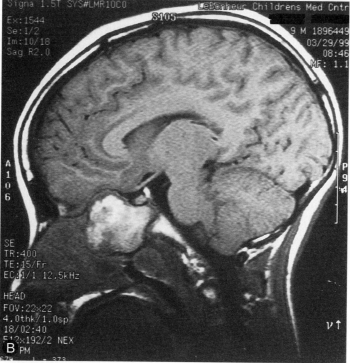

FIGURE 6-8

Allergic fungal sinusitis, eroding the skull base: **A,** computed tomography scan; **B,** magnetic resonance image.

Nasal Cultures. The most common pathogens in chronic sinus infections are well known. In the vast majority of cases, the infection is polymicrobial and anaerobic organisms are nearly always involved. Empiric antibiotic therapy is usually effective. Therefore, cultures are not necessary in most cases. However, when initial antibiotic therapy fails or when atypical pathogens are suspected, a valid culture can be used to guide therapy. Cultures from intranasal swabs are not helpful, because the results correlate poorly with the pathogens in a sinus infection. The traditionally accepted gold standard for culture in sinusitis is to obtain by maxillary sinus lavage. Moreover, if the maxillary sinus is filled with pus that does not drain, the lavage may be therapeutic as well as diagnostic. However, the maxillary antrum is not involved in every case of sinusitis. An alternative source for a culture sample is pus drained from the middle or superior meatus. This is most effectively accessed under endoscopic guidance, using topical anesthesia and vasoconstriction.

Ciliary Dyskinesia. When chronic bacterial sinusitis persists despite aggressive management, the patient may have a ciliary dyskinesia, which impairs mucus clearance, or immunodeficiency. Mucociliary clearance can be easily tested in the clinic. A drop of saccharine is place on the middle turbinate, and the patient is instructed not to sniff. A sweet taste should be detected within 5–8 minutes. Twelve minutes is considered slow, and 25 minutes or longer indicates a mucociliary transport disorder. Nasal mucosal biopsy, analyzed by electron microscopy, can detect whether this is due to a structural abnormality of cilia. Of course, at present there is no specific therapy to correct primary ciliary dyskinesia, and treatment is directed at only mitigating its effects. Thus, the cost of electron microscopy may not be justified.

Immunodeficiency. Immunodeficiency may play a role in chronic or recurrent infection and should be suspected in recalcitrant disease with normal mucosal clearance or in patients with unusual pathogens or a family history of immunodeficiency. If recurrent infections are bacterial and antibody deficiency may be involved, most commonly an immunoglobulin subclass deficiency. Both antibody levels and functional response should be tested.

Natural History

Chronic sinusitis is one of the most common illnesses in the United States, affecting approximately 15% of the population. Some patients have symptoms are constant and indolent, whereas others experience intermittent flare-ups of acute infection.

Significant pain may represent development of a mucocele, which results from the buildup of pressure with an occluded sinus. This pressure can result in gradual expansion of the sinus. Mucoceles may

CRITERIA FOR DIAGNOSING CHRONIC SINUSITIS

Temporal Criteria

> 12 weeks

Clinical Factors

Major:
- Facial pain/pressure
- Facial congestion/fullness
- Nasal obstruction/blockage
- Nasal discharge/purulence/discolored postnasal drip
- Decreased or absent sense of smell

Minor:
- Headache
- Fever
- Halitosis
- Fatigue
- Dental pain
- Cough
- Ear pressure/fullness

Clinical Certainty

Strong:
- ≥ 2 major factors
  - or
- 1 major + 2 minor factors
  - or
- Nasal purulence on examination

Suggestive:
- Major factor
  - or
- ≥ 2 minor factors

---

be the result of chronic infection or to scarring due to trauma or surgery. An infected mucocele is a mucopyocele. Mucoceles usually occur in the ethmoid or frontal sinuses and can present as proptosis. In the sphenoid, a mucocele presents as visual disturbance or as severe headache, usually in the vertex of the skull.

Pott's puffy tumor is a subcutaneous abscess resulting from erosion of infection through the anterior wall of the frontal sinus. Chronic sinusitis may also result in periorbital cellulitis or abscess. Such an infection can lead to osteomyelitis.

Intracranial infections are the most serious sequelae of chronic sinusitis and should be suspected in patients with severe headache, neurologic signs, or fever. An epidural abscess is an indolent process, whereas a subdural abscess results in a rapid downhill course. An intracerebral abscess may produce very minimal symptoms until the abscess ruptures, which is a catastrophic event. Cavernous sinus thrombosis presents as chemosis and ocular nerve palsy and is usually fatal.

Treatment

Many cases of chronic sinusitis are the result of inadequate treatment of acute sinusitis. Therefore, the first step in management is to ensure that the patient has had an optimal course of appropriate antimicrobial therapy. Medical treatment of chronic sinusitis requires a longer course of therapy with drugs active against the relatively resistant organisms that are present. Chronic sinusitis usually involves a mixed infection; anaerobic bacteria and staphylococci are common. Cultures, obtained by sinus irrigation or endoscopic suction, are helpful in guiding therapy. Amoxicillin–clavulanate offers excellent coverage of these organisms. If the patient has a penicillin allergy or a gastrointestinal sensitivity to amoxicillin–clavulanate, then cefuroxime or clindamycin should be considered. Topical nasal steroids, and sometimes systemic steroids, should be used to decrease nasal congestion. Antibiotic therapy should be continued for at least 1 month, and frequently for 2 months. Duration is based on the length of time required for resolution of symptoms. If symptoms do not resolve, CT scanning should be performed to determine whether surgical intervention is warranted.

When intensive medical therapy sometimes results in complete resolution of the symptoms, the patient should be examined carefully. Underlying causes of sinusitis, such as polyps or abnormal anatomy, are most easily detected in the absence of edema and inflammation. If the patient has a history of multiple recurrences of sinusitis, evaluation should include CT scanning, to evaluate anatomy and to detect residual sinus opacification. In children, chronic sinusitis is frequently associated with chronic adenoiditis, and adenoidectomy may solve the problem.

When to Refer

Upper respiratory infections such as the common cold are frequent occurrences. However, if the patient reports four or more episodes per year of acute nose and sinus symptoms or has chronic problems that are not adequately controlled by medical management, consultation is needed to establish the nature and cause of the problem so that appropriate therapy can be planned. If the patient has allergic rhinitis, desensitization therapy may be effective in eliminating or reducing the frequency of infections. Polyps, tumors, or anatomic abnormalities of sinus structure are indications for surgical intervention. Patients with recalcitrant chronic or recurrent sinusitis should be evaluated for possible immunodeficiency or ciliary dyskinesia.

Surgery is indicated in the patient who has recalcitrant chronic infection, whose condition is unresponsive to aggressive medical management, and who has identifiable and correctable pathology, as demonstrated by the CT scan and/or nasal endoscopy.

Today, endoscopic sinus surgery has become the standard of care in most cases. Long-term results are better and perioperative morbidity is greatly reduced in comparison to older, open techniques of sinus surgery. Telescopes permit precise identification of anatomy and pathology. This eliminates the need for blind exenteration of air cells, reducing the risk of injury to the orbit or intracranial space. Endoscopic surgery focuses on establishing physiologic drainage rather than on exenterating infected mucosa. Additionally, nasal endoscopy permits postoperative inspection and débridement of the surgical bed, reducing the risk of adhesions. Endoscopic surgery is best performed when the patient has been optimally treated medically, to reduce swelling and bleeding and facilitate rapid healing.

Surgery is urgently indicated in patients with intracranial infections and in patients with orbital infections or Pott's puffy tumor whose condition does not respond promptly to medical therapy. In such cases, mucosal swelling and increased bleeding can make endoscopic surgery difficult or impossible, and open procedures may be indicated.

KEY POINTS

— Chronic sinusitis often results from inadequate antibiotic therapy.

— Six to 8 weeks of appropriate antibiotic therapy is often effective.

— Surgery is indicated when medical management fails and correctable pathology is identified.

— Surgery is urgently indicated in patients with severe complications.

Suggested Reading

Anon, JB (guest ed.). Report of the Rhinosinusitis Task Force Committee meeting. *Otolaryngol Head Neck Surg* August 1996.
Gliklich RE, Metson R. Health impact of chronic sinusitis in patients seeking otolaryngologic care. *Otolaryngol Head Neck Surg* 113:104–109, 1995.

Fungal Sinusitis

Fungal involvement of the sinuses occurs in one of three forms: invasive, noninvasive, and allergic.

Invasive fungal sinusitis is a grave condition requiring urgent therapy. It occurs in patients with impaired host defenses due to diabetes, leukemia, immunosuppressive medication, chronic renal failure, or acquired immunodeficiency syndrome. The infection originates in the maxillary or ethmoid sinuses and spreads, eventually involving the orbit and nasal cavity, with ischemia and necrosis. The earliest symptoms are mild and nondiagnostic, but many patients present, in later stages, with blindness, ophthalmoplegia, or facial paralysis. Death results from spread into the brain. Prognosis is improved by early detection and aggressive therapy, including drug therapy, and surgical débridement back to bleeding tissue, sometimes requiring sacrifice of the orbit. An important early physical sign is necrosis of the nasal turbinates, appearing as black or dark red areas. Diagnosis is established when biopsy of the nasal mucosa reveals nonseptate hyphae. In patients with diabetes, the pathogen is usually *Mucor,* because this organism thrives in an acid environment, rich in glucose. *Aspergillus* is another pathogen.

Noninvasive fungal sinusitis is a benign condition in which a sinus is obstructed and colonized by fungi, most commonly *Aspergillus.* Colonization may present as fluid in the sinus or as a mycetoma, or fungus ball. Surgical drainage and débridement is generally sufficient treatment.

Allergic fungal sinusitis is generally diagnosed intraoperatively in patients with recalcitrant chronic sinusitis. It may be suspected preoperatively on the basis of findings of calcified foci or CT scanning (Fig. 6–9). The sinuses contain thick and viscous secretions populated by dematiaceous fungi, such *Aspergillus, Helminthosporium, Alternaria,* and *Bipolaris.* This is not a true infection and the patients are not immunocompromised. The fundamental problem is intense allergy to fungi in the atmosphere. The process can result in expansion of the sinus cavities, sometimes presenting as proptosis. Management should include surgery, local and systemic steroids, and allergy control. Antifungal medication is not generally required.

Pediatric Rhinosinusitis

The management of rhinosinusitis differs somewhat in infants and children, because of changes in the anatomy of sinuses during development. At birth, the maxillary and ethmoid sinuses are present but minuscule. The maxillary sinus is only a slitlike cavity running beside the middle turbinate. Because the sinuses are small and insufficient, clinical sinusitis is quite rare the first years of life.

The maxillary sinus gradually enlarges inferiorly and laterally. Inferior expansion is literally limited by unerupted teeth, and the sinus expands inferiorly as teeth erupt. The frontal sinus appear at age 5 or 6 and are not fully developed until late adolescence. Thus, sinusitis in very young children is usually confined to the ethmoid sinuses. Maxillary sinus irrigation should be used with caution in

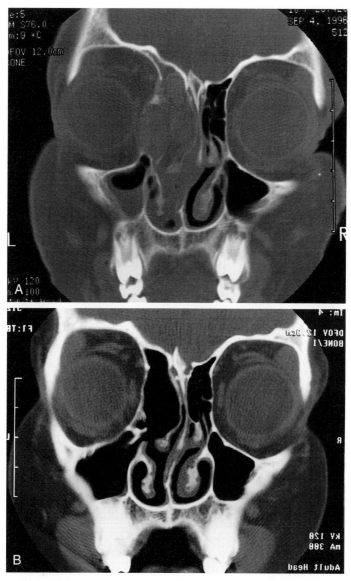

FIGURE 6–9
Computed tomography scan of fungal sinusitis: **A,** before surgery; **B,** after surgery.

children and should not be performed in children younger than 3 years of age, to avoid damage to unerupted teeth.

The clinical presentation of sinusitis in children is often obscure. Many patients present with secondary manifestations, such as cough, epistaxis, mouth breathing, or asthma.

The indications for sinus surgery are much less frequent in children than in adults. Because URIs are so common in young children, recurring sinusitis is rarely an indication for surgery, as similarly, a chronic "runny nose" is more acceptable in a child than in an adult. However, in children with persistent cough, severe asthma, or recurrent epistaxis, sinusitis that does not respond to intensive medical treatment may require surgery. The average pediatrician would be expected to refer one to two patients per year for surgical treatment of chronic sinusitis. Other indications include fungal sinusitis, cystic fibrosis with polyposis, and periorbital abscess.

It should be remembered that purulent rhinorrhea in children is frequently due to adenoiditis and that chronically infected adenoid tissue may serve as a reservoir of pathogens responsible for chronic or recurrent sinusitis. Thus, in a child with chronic rhinitis that is not responsive to medical management, adenoidectomy should be considered a surgical option before resorting to sinus surgery.

Other Nasal Conditions

Rhinitis of Pregnancy. Rhinitis is a common manifestation of pregnancy. It is benign and resolves spontanelusly after delivery. Symptoms generally peak in the third trimester.

Many systemic diseases can cause nasal inflammation and congestion, and some may initially present with such symptoms as nasal obstruction, pain, or epistaxis or with recurrent sinus infection. These disorders should be kept in mind when evaluating patients with chronic nasal complaints.

Sarcoidosis. Sarcoidosis is an idiopathic chronic granulomatous disease, most often affecting the lungs and mediastinal lymph nodes. Occasionally, patients present with nasal obstruction. Nasal mucosa is thickened and inflamed, and there may be significant crusting. Diagnosis is made on the basis of nasal mucosa biopsy or by diagnosis of pulmonary sarcoid.

Treatment is symptomatic. Systemic intralesional injection of steroids may be helpful.

Wegener's Granulomatosis. Wegener's granulomatosis is an uncommon vasculitis affecting the respiratory tract and kidneys. It often presents as chronic rhinitis with crusting, nasal obstruction, and sometimes epistaxis. Early diagnosis is desirable, as the disease, untreated, has a mortality rate of 90% within a few years. Nasal biopsy is usually nondiagnostic, as the subtle vasculitis is obscured by inflammation and necrosis. Diagnosis has been facilitated by the availability of the cytoplasmic antineutrophil cytoplasmic antibody assay.

Cystic Fibrosis. Cystic fibrosis usually manifests itself in early childhood, and lung involvement is usually predominant. However, cystic fibrosis should be suspected in the child with significant chronic sinusitis or polyposis. The onset of polyposis in these patients is typically between the ages of 5 and 14 years. The rate of polyp formation tends to slow in adulthood. Diagnosis of cystic fibrosis is made by sweat chloride test and/or genetic testing. Management of sinus infections in these patients is complicated by the fact that x-rays and

CT scanning are not helpful in detecting infection because the sinuses are generally filled with polyps. Antibiotic therapy should include coverage for *Pseudomonas aeruginosa, H. influenzae, Staphylococcus aureus,* and *Escherichia coli,* too.

Rhinoscleroma. Rhinoscleroma is an infection that is rarely seen in the United States but is endemic to Central and South America and to the Middle East. It presents with purulent nasal discharge and progresses to granulomatous inflammation and fibrotic obstruction of the nose, larynx, trachea, and bronchi. The active stage responds to treatment with streptomycin or tetracycline, but fibrosis is irreversible. Rhinoscleroma should be suspected in immigrants or travelers from endemic areas who have nasal symptoms. Diagnosis is made by culture and by the characteristic histologic appearance on biopsy.

Suggested Readings

Andraca R, Edson RS, Kern EB: Rhinoscleroma: a growing concern in the United States? Mayo Clinic experience. Mayo Clin Proc 68(12):1151–1157, 1993.

deShazo RD, O'Brien MM, Justice WK, Pitcock J: Diagnostic criteria for sarcoidosis of the sinuses. *J Allergy Clin Immunol* 103(5 Pt 1):789–795, 1999.

Ellegard E, Hellgren M, Toren K, Karlsson G: The incidence of pregnancy rhinitis. *Gynecol Obstet Invest* 49(2):98–101, 2000.

Jones NS: Nasal manifestations of rheumatic diseases. *Ann Rheum Dis* 58(10):589–590, 1999.

Nishioka GJ, Cook PR: Paranasal sinus disease in patients with cystic fibrosis. *Otolaryngol Clin North Am* 29(1):193–205, 1996.

7

THE ORAL CAVITY AND THROAT

INTRODUCTION

Sore throat is one of the most common complaints encountered in the general population. Tonsillitis alone has been estimated to account for up to 15% of pediatric office visits. Throat pain may result from a number of inflammatory processes, including infection, allergy, autoimmunity, and gastroesophageal reflux. Although sore throat is most often benign and self-limited, it may also be the initial sign of an impending airway emergency or of a malignant tumor. Inflammatory disorders of the throat may also present with obstructive symptoms of stridor or dysphagia.

Acute Infectious Pharyngitis

It is virtually impossible to distinguish between viral and bacterial throat infections on the basis of findings on clinical examination. Both are manifested by sore throat, fever, odynophagia, and malaise and are often accompanied by cough and lymphadenopathy. Although acute pharyngitis is widely regarded as a streptococcal disease, most cases of the disease are viral. Moreover, although group A β-hemolytic streptococci (GABHS) are very common, they are not the only bacterial pathogens. Recurrent or chronic infections are usually polymicrobial, often including anaerobic organisms.

Most acute throat infections, whether bacterial or viral, are self-limited. Antibiotic therapy is not required for cure but merely hastens recovery and reduces morbidity, and only in that subset of patients who have bacterial infection. Empiric use of antibiotics in all patients with acute pharyngitis cannot be justified, because such treatment is of no benefit in most patients and contributes to the emergence of antimicrobial-resistant strains of bacteria. But the compelling rationale for antibiotic therapy in patients with acute pharyngitis (who do not have a history of recurrent infection) is to prevent the severe sequelae of streptococcal infection, including rheumatic fever and glomerulonephritis. Thus, an ideal clinical protocol for acute pharyngitis would correctly identify and adequately treat all cases of streptococcal pharyngitis while avoiding unnecessary antibiotics.

Diagnosis

Clinical examination of the pharynx is unreliable in distinguishing between viral and bacterial tonsillitis and in determining the need for antibiotic therapy. Both present with erythematous and swollen tonsils, which may be covered by a diffuse exudate or have discharge emanating from the crypts. Fever and lymphadenopathy are signs of both types of infection. Infectious mononucleosis should be suspected if there is diffuse adenopathy or involvement of the liver and spleen. Because of this, the physical examination should always include an abdominal examination.

Throat culture is widely regarded as the gold standard for establishing the cause of tonsillitis. In practice, cultures are widely performed but rarely employed in treatment decisions. More than 30 million throat cultures are ordered in the United States each year. In most cases, treatment is instituted before results are available, and treatment is usually not terminated if the culture results are negative.

Strep antigen detection tests can provide rapid results, with a sensitivity in the range of 80% and a specificity of around 90%. These tests involve extraction of strep antigen and detection with an antibody-tagged label. The test should be performed immediately, or as soon as possible, because accuracy diminishes as the interval between sampling and testing increases.

If the strep test results are negative but clinical suspicion of streptococcal infection is strong, a culture should be used to confirm the result. Cultures obtained from swabs of the palate, buccal mucosa, or pharynx are less reliable indicators of pathogens than samples taken from the tonsil itself.

Discriminate scoring systems have been described with the intent of enhancing the specificity of the clinical examination in detecting infection by GABHS. The Breese scoring system was developed for use in children but requires a white blood cell (WBC) count for every patient. The Walsh system, developed for use in adults, is derived

BREESE STREPTOCOCCAL SCORING SYSTEM FOR CHILDREN

Months	Score	Age (Years)	Score	White Blood Cell Count	Score	Symptoms and Signs	Yes	No	?
Feb, Mar, Apr	4	5–10	4	8–8.4	1	Temperature >100.5°F	4	2	2
Jan, May, Dec	3	4, 11–14	3	8.5–10.4	2	Sore throat	4	2	2
June, Oct, Nov	2	3 or > 15	2	10.5–13.4	3	Cough	2	4	4
July, Aug, Sept	1	≤2	1	13.5–20.4	5	Headache	4	2	2
				≥20.5	6	↑ Nodes	4	2	3
				Not done	3	Abnormal Pharnx	4	1	3

Total Score	Risk of Group A β-Hemolytic Streptococci
≤ 25	6%
25–31	50%
32–38	84%

from characteristics of the history and physical examination. Use of such protocols avoids the costs of culture and antibiotic treatment in some patients, with very little risk of failure to treat those infections with a potential to cause rheumatic fever. For example, adult patients with a Walsh score of ≤ 30 have a less than 20% chance of having GABHS, whereas nearly 100% of patients with a score > 40 have GABHS.

Other conditions should be considered. Patients with severe tonsillitis and lymphadenopathy may have infectious mononucleosis. Diagnosis is established by the laboratory findings of lymphocytosis with atypical lymphocytes and by positive heterophile antibody testing. Coxsackievirus infection results in severe throat pain, with a vesicular eruption of the mucosa of the tonsils, pharynx, and palate. Another condition to be considered in the differential of acute tonsillitis is diphtheria. Diphtheria is rare in the United States, owing to widespread immunization, but sporadic cases occur. A characteristic "wet mouse" odor has been classically associated with this disease. The characteristic sign on physical examination is a gray membrane, firmly adherent to the pharyngeal mucosa. This membrane may enlarge, resulting in airway obstruction. Toxins released systemically can result in circulatory collapse. Antibiotics are useful only as adjuvant therapy, and definitive treatment requires antitoxin.

Natural History

Most cases of acute pharyngitis are benign and self-limited. However, severe complications can result from tonsillitis. Acute tonsillar swelling can obstruct the airway. Local spread of infection can result in peritonsillar abscess. Streptococcal infection can result in rheumatic fever, a serious immune-mediated disease composed of arthritis, heart disease, and/or chorea. Another immune-mediated consequence of streptococcal infection is acute glomerulonephritis. Scarlet fever is caused by an erythrogenic toxin released by streptococci. A red punctate rash appears on the second day of the infection and lasts about 1 week, desquamation follows. The rash initially involves the trunk, spreading to nearly the entire body within hours. The tongue has a characteristic strawberry appearance. Persistent changes in the tonsil after an acute infection can make it more susceptible to repeated infections.

Treatment

Penicillin has long been regarded as the drug of choice for streptococcal pharyngitis. Oral administration is just as effective as intramuscular injection, provided patients complete the course of therapy. The American Heart Association recommends a 10-day regimen of oral penicillin V, 250 mg three times per day. Some sources recommend a dose of 500 mg three times per day, in adults and children older than 12. Erythromycin is the recommended alternative antibiotic for patients who are allergic to penicillin. Prompt treatment is not essential for the prevention of rheumatic fever, as penicillin therapy is effective even when instituted as late as 9 days after onset of symptoms.

Other medications with broader spectra, such as amoxicillin (with or without clavulanate), cephalosporins, clindamycin, and newer macrolides, are as effective as penicillin, and some studies suggest they have greater efficacy. The reports of decreasing effectiveness of penicillin and the emergence of resistant strains could be interpreted as support for the use of broad-spectrum antibiotics in the treatment of acute streptococcal pharyngitis and the prevention of post-streptococcal complications. However, despite the reports that penicillin efficacy is diminishing, there has been no corresponding increase in the incidence of rheumatic fever in patients whose disease is managed with penicillin. One possible explanation for this could be that the strains of Streptococcus that result in rheumatic fever have not become penicillin resistant. Whatever the reason, penicillin still seems effective in preventing rheumatic complications, and unnecessary use of broad-spectrum antibiotics could contribute to problems of drug resistance.

Streptococcal pharyngitis generally resolves within 5 days, with or without antibiotics. When recovery does not occur within this time frame, the diagnosis of streptococcal infection should be questioned. Other bacteria may be involved, particularly if the patient has had previous episodes of tonsillitis. Another cause of persisting symptoms is the development of peritonsillar abscess or cellulitis. The possibility of infectious mononucleosis should be explored with blood tests and examination for systemic signs of the disease. Acute onset of pharyngeal inflammation may be the presenting sign of an uncommon mucosal disorder, such as pemphigus, pemphigoid, or giant aphthous ulcerations.

When to Refer

Significant airway distress in any patient warrants an otolaryngologic consultation. Acute onset of severe sore throat with dyspnea and dysphagia could represent epiglottitis, a condition that can be rapidly fatal without appropriate airway management. In other cases, stridor may be due to acute enlargement of tonsils. Patients suspected of having peritonsillar infection generally require otolaryngologic evaluation. Sore throat that does not resolve within 2 weeks is a potential indication for endoscopic evaluation of the nasopharynx, hypopharynx, and larynx. Patients with recalcitrant tonsillitis should be considered as candidates for tonsillectomy.

KEY POINTS

— A viral infection cannot be distinguished from a bacterial infection on physical examination.

— Rapid strep testing and clinical scoring systems are useful in identification of patients who will benefit from antibiotic therapy.

— Penicillin therapy is adequate for prevention of autoimmune complications of streptococcal infection.

— Otolaryngologic consultation is advisable for patients with airway compromise or with sore throat lasting more than 2 weeks.

Suggested Readings

Breese BB. A simple coregard for the tentative diagnosis of streptococcal pharyngitis. *Am J Dis Child* 131:514–517, 1977.
Pichichere ME. Group A beta-hemolytic streptococcal pharyngitis. In Johnson JT, Yu VL: *Infectious Diseases and Antimicrobial Therapy of the Ears, Nose, and Throat.* Philadelphia: WB Saunders, 1997, pp 406–421.
Walsh BT, Brookheim WW, Johnson RC, et al. Recognition of streptococcal pharyngitis in adults. *Arch Intern Med* 135:1493–1497, 1975.

Recurrent and Chronic Tonsillitis

One tonsil infection once every few years does not constitute recurrent tonsillitis. Patients with chronic or recurrent tonsillitis are those in whom repeated or prolonged infection has diminished the capacity of the tonsil to fight infection. This results in a chronically infected tonsil or continual recrudescences of acute infection. Presenting symptoms include frequent or constant sore throat, halitosis, and dysphagia. Antibiotics usually provide varying durations and degrees of improvement. Commonly, chronic and recurrent infections lead to lymphoid hyperplasia, with enlargement of the tonsil. Enlargement may be sufficient to result in obstructive sleep apnea. However, in many cases, prolonged or repeated infection results in a small and scarred tonsil. Chronic tonsillitis may occur as the aftermath of infectious mononucleosis.

The histologic changes associated with chronic tonsillitis are quite significant. The normal tonsil contains lymphoid follicles and 10–20 deep crypts in the surface that serve as collection and processing sites for inhaled and ingested antigens and pathogens. The epithelial lining of the crypts contains micropore (M) cells, which are tubuvesicular in structure and facilitate entry of antigens into the tonsil. With increasing infection exposure, the epithelium of the crypts also undergoes squamous metaplasia and loss of M cells. These changes decrease the immune capacity of the tonsil, and leading to a tolerance for bacteria in the crypts. The metaplasia also results in a buildup of desquamated debris in the crypts. This retained debris is fertile grounds for chronic bacterial infection and is particularly conducive to anaerobic organisms.

In its extreme form, squamous metaplasia results in "cryptic tonsillitis," with frequent discharge of cheesy, malodorous discharge into the mouth. The squamous debris may organize into firm, rocklike particles, termed tonsilloliths. Some patients may not experience sore throats, but find their social and work interactions significantly impaired by the continual halitosis and foul-smelling discharge. Frequently, patients report their own attempts to keep the tonsils clean, using cotton-tipped applicators or digital pressure to express debris from the tonsils.

Diagnosis

A history of chronic or repeated episodes of sore throat is not sufficient for the diagnosis of tonsillitis. Throat pain may result from a variety of causes, including sinusitis, gastroesophageal reflux, laryngeal arthritis, cervical osteophytes, and temporomandibular joint disorders. Physical examination can detect the changes of chronic or repeated infections. Tonsils may be enlarged, normal-size, or small. Deep and enlarged crypts are frequently seen, often filled with food particles and squamous debris. But in patients with recurrent infections, the tonsils may appear normal between acute episodes, and the size of the tonsil does not correlate with the severity of the problem. Thus, the diagnosis of recurrent tonsillitis must be established on the basis of physical examination during an acute episode. Cervical lymphadenopathy is common, with shoddy nodes that become enlarged and tender during acute exacerbations of infection. In children, the adenoids are usually also involved in the infectious process, resulting in nasal obstruction and sometimes purulent nasal discharge. Otitis media is also a common accompanying problem in children.

Cultures are not necessary for the diagnosis of chronic and recurrent tonsillitis and are usually not helpful in planning therapy.

Natural History

Patients usually report repeated or constant sore throat over the course of several months. Often there is an escalating pattern of severity and decreasing duration of asymptomatic intervals. In other patients, the throat is constantly sore, but the soreness may fluctuate in severity. When the infections lead to hypertrophy of the tonsils, obstructive symptoms may predominate. The most common cause of obstructive sleep apnea in children is tonsil or adenoid hypertrophy.

Treatment

Recurrent and chronic tonsillitis is generally a polymicrobial disorder. The fundamental problem is a failure of local host defenses, rather than a bacterial disease that satisfies Koch's postulates. Management therefore includes not only broad-spectrum antibiotics to decrease the bacteria population of the tonsil but also local measures to reduce stasis in the tonsillar crypts.

Studies based on cultures from the surface or core of the tonsils indicate five different pathogens per patient, with a high incidence of anaerobic bacteria and a high incidence of B-lactamase–producing organisms. Empiric antibiotic therapy based on this information requires prolonged therapy with a broad-spectrum antibiotic, with good coverage of anaerobic organisms. For most patients, amoxicillin with clavulanate is optimal. Cefuroxime is also an excellent choice, particularly in patients who experience gastrointestinal side effects from amoxicillin–clavulanate.

Treatment of chronic and recurrent tonsillitis should continue for 6–8 weeks. A shorter duration can leave a significant population of bacteria within the crypts. Moreover, tonsils may remain swollen for several weeks after resolution of an acute infection and therefore will be susceptible to recurrent infection.

Once edema has resolved, local cleaning of the tonsils can reduce stasis within the crypts. This decreases halitosis and reduces the incidence of repeat infections. Gentle daily cleaning of the tonsils is recommended, using a pulsed water irrigation device, designed for oral hygiene (e.g., Water Pik). This can be done using salt water or a dilute solution of mouthwash and/or hydrogen peroxide.

If medical treatment fails, tonsillectomy should be considered. Tonsillectomy is indicated when the morbidity of tonsil infections outweighs the risks and cost of surgery. This is ideally a personal decision between the patient (or the patient's parents) and the surgeon. But in today's third-party payer environment, rigid criteria have been developed. In most protocols, a patient who has had four or more infections within 1 year or fewer infections per year for several years is a candidate for tonsillectomy. Fewer episodes are required if infection was "severe."

Criteria for a rating of "severe" include episodes that cause a loss of more than 5 days from work or school, airway obstruction, peritonsillar abscess, or hospitalization. Tonsillectomy is also indicated for local hygiene in patients with significant intraoral discharge of crypt contents.

Some decision trees for tonsillectomy require culture or rapid strep test documentation of recurrent streptococcal infection. This is not a valid parameter, because, as discussed above, recurrent infections may involve a variety of organisms.

Postoperatively, patients experience varying degrees of throat pain and dysphagia. In some cases, patients may not be able to swallow even liquids for 1 or 2 days. Nasal regurgitation during swallowing is common during the first few days. Halitosis and pain can be significantly reduced by routine administration of postoperative antibiotics. Resumption of a normal diet often requires 2 to 3 weeks.

Complications have been reported to occur in between 1% and 5% of tonsillectomies. Postoperative bleeding is the most common problem, characteristically occurring either within 24 hours of surgery or about 1 week later, when the eschar detaches from the surgical bed. This sometimes resolves spontaneously or can be managed by local measures. However, postoperative bleeding is sometimes fatal. Although this is a rare occurrence, diligence requires that any patient with significant bleeding should be taken back to the operating room for exploration and control of the bleeding under general anesthesia. Postobstructive pulmonary edema may occur immediately after surgery or within several hours and may be fatal. Treatment requires prompt initiation of positive-pressure ventilation. Other complications of tonsillectomy are rare.

The mouth gag suspension system commonly used in tonsillectomy and adenoidectomy requires hyperextension of the neck. This can dislocate an unstable atlantoaxial joint, resulting in quadriplegia. As many as 10% of those affected with Down syndrome have laxity of the atlantoaxial joint. Quadriplegia has never been reported as a complication of tonsillectomy in a patient with Down syndrome; nonetheless, surgery should be approached with caution in this population, with preoperative evaluation of the cervical spine.

Opinions vary in regard to whether tonsillectomy should be performed on an inpatient or outpatient basis. Most children and many adults can be discharged on the same day. However, a longer stay may be required if the patient cannot maintain an adequate oral

INDICATIONS FOR TONSILLECTOMY

Three or more infections per year
Hypertrophy causing:
  Dental malocclusion
  Facial growth impairment
  Upper airway obstruction
  Sleep disorders
  Cardiopulmonary complications
  Severe dysphagia
Peritonsillar abscess
Persistent foul taste due to chronic infection
Chronic tonsillitis in a streptococcal carrier
Unilateral hypertrophy, suspected neoplasia

(Adapted from 1998 Compendium of Clinical Indicators. American Academy of Otolaryngology, Alexandria, VA)

intake or if there is significant oozing from the tonsillar bed after surgery. Planned overnight admission is recommended for children under the age of 3 years, because of a higher risk of postoperative complications. Additionally, any patient with significant upper airway obstruction should be watched overnight for potential onset of postobstructive pulmonary edema.

Lingual tonsils may become enlarged or chronically infected, months or years after removal of the palatine tonsils. The lingual tonsils are ill-defined collections of lymphoid tissue on the lingual surface of the vallecula and are a part of Waldeyer's tonsillar ring. This tissue is not removed as a part of standard tonsillectomy and is clinically insignificant in most patients. But in some patients, chronic infection and hypertrophy of lingual tonsil tissue results in chronic sore throat, dysphagia, and, in some cases, upper airway obstruction. A 6-week course of antibiotic therapy, including anaerobic coverage, may result in resolution, but surgical removal is usually required.

Suggested Readings

Paradise JL, Bluestone CE, Bachman RZ, et al. Efficacy of tonsillectomy for recurrent throat infection in severely affected children: Results of parallel randomized and non-randomized clinical trials. N Engl J Med 310:674–683, 1984.
Scadding GK. Immunology of the tonsil: A review. J Roy Soc Med 83:104–107, 1990.

Peritonsillar Abscess (Quinsy)

Peritonsillar abscess is a common problem, with an annual incidence in the United States of about 30 per 100,000 people. It most often occurs in adolescents and young adults but is also seen in younger and older patients. Most patients report a preceding throat infection, but some do not. Patients who have one peritonsillar abscess are at increased risk for a second or third. Recurrence is more likely in patients with a history of recurrent tonsillitis, particularly those younger than 30 years of age.

Peritonsillar abscess is a complication of tonsillitis. Antibiotic treatment of tonsillitis does not prevent abscess formation, as more than half of patients who have peritonsillar abscess are taking antibiotics at the time of presentation. Symptoms of peritonsillar abscess include sore throat, dysphagia, trismus, and fever. The voice sounds muffled, with a characteristic "hot potato" voice. Symptoms progress gradually, so that most patients present 3–5 days after disease onset.

Diagnosis

Severe sore throat and dysphagia should raise the suspicion of peritonsillar abscess. Diagnosis is based on findings on physical examination of the mouth, to distinguish severe tonsillitis from peritonsillar abscess or cellulitis. On the involved side, the tonsil is displaced medially and the soft palate bulges above the tonsil. The uvula frequently deviates to the side opposite the abscess (Fig. 7–1). Visualiza-

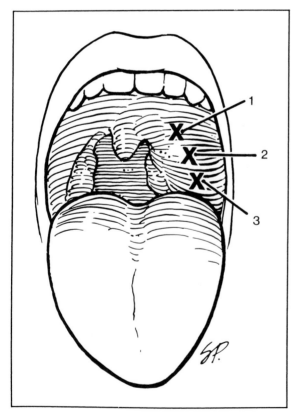

FIGURE 7–1
Peritonsillar abscess: recommended points for needle aspiration.

tion of the posterior pharynx is sometimes quite dif
edema of the soft palate and to trismus, which limits
jaw. Trismus can be relieved by the use of topical
ipsilateral middle meatus of the nose to produce a s
block (Fig. 7–2).

When characteristic physical signs are present, the existence of
peritonsillar infection is clear. However, it is difficult to differentiate
peritonsillar abscess and cellulitis. Gentle tapping on the mucosa
above the tonsil elicits sharp pain when an abscess is present. However, the diagnosis is conclusively established only when pus is aspirated or drained from the space. Thus, the diagnostic procedure is
usually therapeutic.

Laboratory tests are not needed in routine management of peritonsillar abscess. However, if a patient appears to be dehydrated,
blood chemistry should be evaluated. Cultures of the pus are usually
obtained but not used, because failures are rarely encountered with
the immediate empiric use of antibiotics. This is probably because of
the fact that the drainage itself is the most important determinant
of outcome.

Radiography is unnecessary in the vast majority of patients,
but computed tomography (CT) is quite helpful in some patients.
Computed tomography should be used in patients with asymmetric
tonsil enlargement who do not have fever or other signs of enlargement, as this presentation suggests a tumor or, more rarely, an internal carotid artery aneurysm. Computed tomography is also helpful
in patients who cannot be adequately examined, such as those with
severe trismus, or small children. Finally, when no pus can be ob-

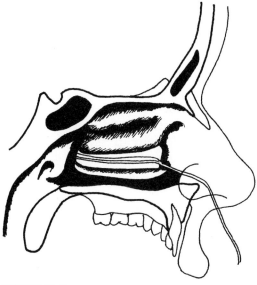

FIGURE 7–2

Technique of sphenopalatine block, to relieve trismus for intraoral examination. A pledget
soaked in 4% cocaine or xylocaine is placed under the middle turbinate.

Gradual onset of severe sore throat
Dysphagia or drooling
Fever
Trismus
Bulging of the tonsil and/or palate with or without deviation of the uvula

tained by needle aspiration but findings on clinical evaluation are highly suggestive of abscess, CT may demonstrate a collection of pus, particularly when the abscess is located in the inferior pole.

Natural History

Untreated peritonsillar abscess produces escalating pain, usually ruptures spontaneously and eventually resolves. The draining pus may be aspirated into the lungs, leading to airway obstruction or pneumonia. An alternate outcome is spread of the infection into the adjacent parapharyngeal space.

Treatment

Traditional treatment of peritonsillar abscess is incision and drainage, under local anesthesia. However, needle aspiration has proven to be equally effective. Three-point aspiration should be performed (Fig. 7–1). General anesthesia is required in very young or otherwise uncooperative patients. If the patient is dehydrated or still unable to swallow after drainage of the abscess, hospital admission is indicated for fluid replacement.

Drainage is generally sufficient treatment for the abscess, but antibiotic therapy is indicated for the accompanying tonsillitis, covering for β-hemolytic streptococci, *Staphylococcus aureus,* and anaerobic organisms. Either penicillin or amoxicillin with clavulanate, given for at least 1 week, is a good choice. Patients should be reevaluated within 24 hours, because the abscess will recur in as many as 15% of patients. Recurrences almost always respond to a second drainage. The few patients whose condition does not resolve after a second drainage should have a tonsillectomy.

Immediate tonsillectomy ("quinsy tonsillectomy") is a treatment option that involves more immediate morbidity than simple drainage; however, it is a sensible choice in patients who have a history of chronic or recurrent tonsillitis. Most of these would be candidates for tonsillectomy even in the absence of the present abscess. It is also recommended for patients aged 30 years or less, because they have an increased risk of a second peritonsillar abscess. The overall morbid-

A TREATMENT STRATEGY

> Drainage by needle aspiration or open incision
> Examination after 24 hours; drain recurrent abscess
> Continued abscess → tonsillectomy
> Exceptions—immediate or interval tonsillectomy if:
>   Age less than 30 years and
>   History of recurrent tonsillitis or prior abscess

ity and time in the hospital is significantly less for patients undergoing immediate tonsillectomy for peritonsillar abscess than for those who have simple drainage and then a tonsillectomy after an interval for recovery.

Suggested Readings

Herzon FS. Peritonsillar abscess: Incidence, current management practices, and a proposal for treatment guidelines. *Laryngoscope* 105(suppl 74):1–17, 1995.

Kronenberg J, Wolf M, Leventon G. Peritonsillar abscess: Recurrence rate and the indication for tonsillectomy. *Am J Otolaryngol* 8:82–84, 1987.

Spires JR, Ownes JJ, Woodson GE, et al. Treatment of peritonsillar abscess: A prospective study of aspiration vs incision and drainage. *Arch Otolaryngol Head Neck Surg* 113:984–986, 1987.

Epiglottitis (Supraglottitis)

Acute infection of the epiglottis and surrounding supraglottic tissue is a clinical emergency because fatal airway obstruction may result. Patients present with fever, throat pain, toxemia, and rapidly progressive stridor. To maintain ventilation, patients typically assume a "sniff" posture, leaning forward with the head extended. Patients may drool and generally avoid lying down. The voice has a characteristic "hot potato" sound, because the swollen epiglottis occupies a large space and alters resonance of the vocal tract. The disease may be indolent in adults, with a prodromal upper respiratory infection (URI), and specific signs of epiglottiditis may develop over a few days. Onset and progression are more rapid in young children. In either age group, early diagnosis and an established protocol are required for optimal outcome.

The most common organism responsible for supraglottitis is *Haemophilus influenzae* type B, although other organisms are frequently implicated in adult infections. The incidence of supraglottitis in adults is fewer than 2 cases per 100,000 people per year. The vast majority of cases occur in children between the ages of 2 and 4 years, and since the introduction of the *H. influenzae* vaccination, the incidence of supraglottiditis has significantly diminished.

Diagnosis

Supraglottitis should be suspected whenever a patient presents with characteristic symptoms of rapid onset of sore throat, fever, and airway distress. Assurance of a stable airway always takes precedence over establishment of a definitive diagnosis. Patients with significant airway distress should be immediately taken to the operating room for emergency intubation or tracheotomy. The diagnosis can be established *after* the airway is secured.

When airway involvement is not severe and the diagnosis is not certain, examination by flexible nasopharyngoscopy is indicated. Topical anesthesia should be used and the examination should be performed very carefully, particularly in children, because choking or gagging could lead to sudden fatal airway occlusion. Intraoral examination usually is not helpful, as the posterior pharyngeal wall is not involved. Further, depression of the tongue with a tongue blade may also lead to airway obstruction. Palpation usually reveals tenderness above the "Adam's apple," in the region of the thyrohyoid membrane.

If the epiglottis cannot be visualized and the airway is not significantly compromised, a soft-tissue lateral x-ray of the neck is indicated. The swollen epiglottis results in a characteristic "thumbprint sign" (Fig. 7–3). It should be emphasized that x-rays are usually not indicated and should be performed only when the airway is not compromised. Further, a patient suspected of having epiglottitis should never be sent to the radiology department unless accompanied by a physi-

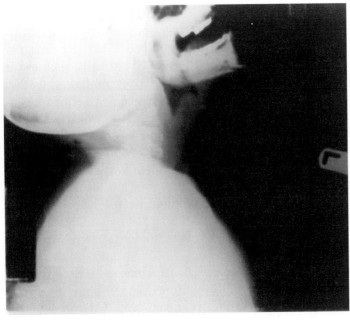

FIGURE 7–3
Lateral soft-tissue film showing epiglottitis.

cian who is capable of emergency airway management and has the necessary equipment available to perform either rapid intubation or an emergency tracheotomy.

The WBC count is significantly elevated in most patients. However, the degree of leukocytosis does not correlate with severity of the disease; therefore, this test is of little or no use.

Cultures are not required to establish the diagnosis but are often important in determining the best antibiotic therapy. Blood culture findings are positive in a large percentage of children and the results correlate well with the pathogens of the supraglottitis. By contrast, mucosal cultures, even from the epiglottis itself, indicate the pathogen in only about 20% of patients. Blood cultures are less reliable in adults.

Natural History

The clinical course in children differs significantly from that in adults. Symptom progression is most rapid in young children, with development of obstruction usually within 12 hours. The disease is more indolent in adults, who generally have a prodromal URI and develop specific signs of epiglottitis over a few days. The severity of airway obstruction appears to be related to the time course of symptom development. The airway is not always significantly compromised in patients with an indolent course. However, the clinical course is unpredictable, as sudden fatal airway obstruction can occur in any patient.

Postobstructive edema may occur after the airway is established. The mechanism of this complication is unknown. Adult respiratory distress syndrome is another possible complication.

Epiglottic abscess is a common complication of epiglottitis in adults. The abscess may be detected during initial laryngoscopy or may only be suspected if the airway does not improve with appropriate antibiotic therapy. The abscess responds well to incision and drainage.

Other sites in the body may become involved by the infection. When the causitive organism is *H. influenzae,* there is a risk of associated meningitis. This is fortunately not a common occurrence, but the combination has a high mortality rate. Thus, it is important to be alert for signs of meningeal irritation. In patients with nucchal rigidity, it is prudent to perform a lumbar puncture, after the airway is secured. Other associated infections include pneumonia and empyema.

Treatment

Establishment of a stable airway is the primary therapeutic objective. In children, this is almost always achieved by endotracheal intubation. A patient with an endotracheal tube must be monitored in an intensive care unit, with immediate availability of personnel to reinsert the tube, should it become dislodged. Endotracheal intubation requires sedation, and often neuromuscular paralysis and mechanical ventilation are also required. The duration of intubation is approximately 2 days, but it may be longer.

Disease management differs somewhat in adults, owing to the more indolent course of the disease and to the logistics of maintaining endotracheal intubation. Although intubation is used widely, there are some advantages to the use of tracheotomy in adults. A tracheotomy is more comfortable in the short run, as it eliminates the need for sedation and restraint and allows patients to eat and often even speak. The tracheotomy tube can be removed in 4–10 days. Some sources advocate watchful waiting in adult patients who present without significant stridor; however, other authors report mortality rates of around 10% for this approach. Patients without significant stridor or who do not assume an upright posture to maintain the airway are reported to have a lesser chance of airway failure. If a choice is made not to use tracheotomy or intubation, then that patient should be monitored extremely closely, with immediate availability of airway intervention, should the situation deteriorate rapidly.

In children, antibiotic therapy should cover *H. influenzae* type B, the most common organism in that age group. In adults, therapy should also include coverage for gram-positive and anaerobic organisms. Because of emerging strains of resistant organisms and the life-threatening nature of this disease, such first-line agents as ampicillin are no longer recommended. Second- or third-generation cephalosporins are currently accepted as appropriate agents. In particular, cefuroxime is widely recommended. Adequate therapy requires a 10-day course of therapy.

When to Refer

Suspected epiglottitis in any patient should be managed by a team that includes an anesthesiologist or critical care physician and an otolaryngologist.

KEY POINTS

— Epiglottitis is an emergency, requiring prompt team management by an established protocol.

— The first priority is establishment of an airway, preferably in the operating room with a surgeon and anesthesiologist present.

— Neck radiographs are not required for diagnosis and are rarely indicated.

— Antibiotic therapy should include coverage for *H. influenzae* as well as for gram-positive and anaerobic organisms.

Suggested Readings

Gorelick MH, Baker MD. Epiglottitis in children, 1979 through 1992: effects of *Haemophilus influenzae* type B immunization. *Arch Pediatr Adolesc Med* 148:47–50, 1994.

MayoSmith MF, Hirsch PH, Wodzinski SF, et al. Acute epiglottitis in adults, an eight-year experience in the state of Rhode Island. *N Engl J Med* 314:1133–1139, 1986.

Croup

Croup is acute airway obstruction due to laryngotracheobronchitis. It is manifested by inspiratory or biphasic high-pitched stridor and a dry, barking cough. Essentially a pediatric disorder, it is the most common cause of upper airway obstruction in children, but it is rare in adults. This age relationship can be attributed to the smaller airway diameter in very young children. Although the inflammation is a diffuse lower airway process, the actual site of airflow restriction is the subglottis. This is the most narrow point of the respiratory tract, bounded by the cricoid cartilage, the only complete cartilage ring in the airway. Mucosal edema within this rigid structure compromises its lumen. There are two chief forms of croup, spasmodic (idiopathic) and infectious.

Spasmodic croup is characterized by rapid onset of mild to moderate stridor and barking cough, with onset usually at night. Patients are afebrile. The stridor resolves spontaneously within a few hours, and often responds to steam or cool mist inhalation. Frequently, this is a recurring problem in very young patients.

Viral coup most often results from human parainfluenza virus. Other pathogens include influenza virus, respiratory syncytial virus, and—rarely—measles virus. Viral croup chiefly afflicts children between the ages of 3 months and 3 years. Peak incidence is in late fall or early winter. The infection usually begins in the nose and then moves down to involve the larynx and trachea. Stridor may occur rapidly, within 2 days, or as long as 2 weeks after the onset of symptoms. Fever is mild or absent and patients do not appear toxic. Bacterial croup is more severe, usually involving high fever and systemic toxicity. It is generally considered to result from bacterial superinfection of viral croup.

Diagnosis

Diagnosis is established by the findings on medical history and physical examination, noting the onset of the characteristic stridor and barking cough and ruling out other causes of airway obstruction, such as epiglottitis, retropharyngeal abscess, or foreign body. High fever, systemic toxicity, and drooling are not consistent with a diagnosis of croup and instead suggest a more severe inflammatory process, such as epiglottitis, or retropharyngeal abscess. Parents should be carefully questioned about possible ingestion of a foreign body, which could be lodged in either the respiratory tract or the esophagus. The bark of croup is generally worse than its bite. Children with croup often seem to be in little or no distress, despite very loud stridor. By contrast, patients with epiglottitis or retropharyngeal abscess are toxic and may have significant difficulty breathing and/or swallowing, without significant stridor.

The medical history and physical should also establish the severity of the croup and predict the likelihood that airway intervention will become necessary. There are several available systems for assigning a "croup score." Most include consideration of the patient's color, respiratory rate, pulse, and the presence and severity of stridor and retractions. Pulse oximetry and transcutaneous measurement of carbon dioxide are valuable in assessing the patient and monitoring response to treatment. Arterial blood gas determinations are not recommended, as they are likely to exacerbate symptoms by stimulating inspiratory effort.

Croup is radiographically manifested by a characteristic steeple appearance of the subglottic airway on anteroposterior view (Fig. 7–4). Lateral radiographs may also demonstrate subglottic narrowing and can also be used to evaluate the supraglottic airway for the possibility of epiglottitis. X-rays are not necessary for diagnosis and should be used only to confirm or document clinical suspicion. In no circumstance should a patient with airway compromise be sent for x-rays without a physician in attendance. Ideally, any needed x-rays should be obtained within the emergency room, by portable technique.

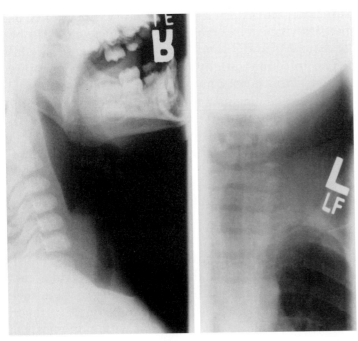

FIGURE 7–4
Radiographic appearance of croup.

Patients whose condition does not respond to medical management may require rigid endoscopy, under general anesthesia, to evaluate and establish the airway. Flexible endoscopy and local anesthesia are not recommended during acute croup, owing to the tenuous nature of the airway. However, elective endoscopy may be indicated between episodes in a patient with recurrent bouts of croup.

SUMMARY OF DIAGNOSTIC SIGNS AND SYMPTOMS
Infants and young children
Stridor and barking, nonproductive cough
Fever mild or absent

Treatment

Spasmodic croup is self-limited, by definition, and steam or cool mist inhalation is frequently helpful in ameliorating or aborting an attack. For children with recurrent spasmodic croup, parents can be instructed in home management of the condition.

Aerosolized racemic epinephrine stimulates adrenergic receptors in the respiratory mucosa, producing vasoconstriction to reduce swelling. This is the initial treatment of choice in hospital management of croup. Rebound congestion is common; therefore, patients should not be discharged immediately after treatment. Monitoring for 1–2 hours is advisable.

Hospital admission is advised for patients with suprasternal or intercostal inspiratory retraction or with significant stridor. Steroids are effective in lessening symptoms and have been statistically demonstrated to reduce the number of cases in which intubation is required. A dose equivalent to 0.3–1 mg/kg dexamethasone is recommended.

Intubation should be considered if the patient appears fatigued or requires supplemental oxygen. It is preferable to establish the airway in the surgical suite, using rigid endoscopy. When medical therapy fails, the patient may have developed membranous bacterial tracheitis, and rigid endoscopy permits removal of obstructing material. It is also possible that the clinical diagnosis of croup is erroneous. The patient could have ingested a foreign body or could have subglottic stenosis or hemangioma. In these problems, orotracheal intubation may be difficult or impossible, with disastrous consequences.

When to Refer

When medical treatment fails or when intubation is considered, specialty consultation is indicated. Rigid endoscopy is usually indicated, to establish the airway and to rule out other causes of airway obstruction.

When patients have recurrent episodes of croup requiring hospitalization, they may have underlying pathology, such as subglottic or tracheal stenosis. Endoscopic evaluation is indicated, preferably on an elective basis, during an asymptomatic interval.

KEY POINTS

— Steroids are effective in viral croup.

— X-rays are usually not needed, but they show the "steeple sign" in the trachea.

— Arterial blood gas determinations are not recommended.

— Hospital admission is indicated for retractions or significant stridor.

Suggested Readings

Cherry JD. Croup. In: Feigin RD, Cherry JD, eds. *Textbook of Pediatric Infectious Disease*, 3rd ed, vol 1. Philadelphia: WB Saunders, 1992, pp 209–220.
Kairys SW, Olmstead EM, O'Connor GT. Steroid treatment of larygotracheitis: A meta-analysis of the evidence from randomized trials. *Pediatrics* 89:302–306, 1992.

Retropharyngeal Abscess

Retropharyngeal abscess in almost exclusively a disease of very young children, as between 71% and 96% of retropharyngeal abscesses occur before the age of 6 years. Up to 50% occur in infants between the ages of 6 and 12 months. Although the retropharyngeal space extends from the base of skull into the mediastinum, abscesses are most often confined to the upper portion. At the second cervical vertebrae, the fascia of the superior constrictor muscle attaches to that of the prevertebral muscles, and this point is often the lower limit of the abscess. Retropharyngeal abscess infections are generally considered to arise from involvement of lymph nodes in the space that drain the sinuses, the pharynx, and the ears. These nodes atrophy after approximately 4 years of age and are not present in adults, which explains the higher incidence of retropharyngeal abscess in young children. Another cause is a penetrating wound of the oropharynx, which may occur when a patient falls with a sharp object in the mouth or may be caused by an ingested sharp object, such as a pin or a fish bone.

Patients characteristically present with fever and dysphagia. A muffled voice, drooling, and a stiff or swollen neck are also common. Many have noisy, stertorous breathing, but significant stridor is not often encountered. A preceding throat or ear infection is common. In fact, the majority of patients with retropharyngeal abscess have been recently treated with antibiotics.

THICKNESS OF PREVERTEBRAL SOFT TISSUE

Level	Child	Adult
C2	< 7 mm	< 7 mm
C6	< 14 mm	< 22 mm

Diagnosis

The pathognomonic physical sign is unilateral fluctuant swelling of the posterior pharyngeal wall. However, physical examination is often difficult, in young children. *Palpation is contraindicated,* as this may cause the abscess to rupture. Thus, diagnosis of retropharyngeal abscess is essentially radiologic. Lateral soft-tissue view of the neck reveals thickening of the prevertebral soft tissue (Fig. 7–5). Other signs that may be apparent on plain films include loss of the normal curvature of the cervical spine and air within an abscess. Computed tomography is more accurate in detecting retropharyngeal infection

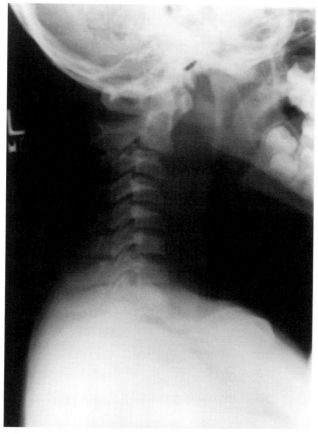

FIGURE 7–5
Radiographic appearance of retropharyngeal abscess.

and is indicated when findings on plain films are equivocal (Fig. 7–6). In the absence of air in the abscess, neither imaging approach reliably differentiates pus from adenitis. If a retropharyngeal abscess is suggested, a chest film is also needed to rule out mediastinitis.

Natural History

Untreated, a retropharyngeal abscess may drain spontaneously and subsequently resolve. However, aspiration of pus can lead to pneumonia or airway obstruction. The infection can also spread into the adjacent parapharyngeal space or through the adjacent danger space into the mediastinum.

Treatment

Patients in whom retropharyngeal abscess has been diagnosed or who are suspected of having it should be admitted to the hospital and treated with intravenous antibiotics. Although surgical drainage is usually needed, the abscess resolves with medical management alone in up to one fourth of patients. Broad-spectrum antibiotics are indicated, including coverage for anaerobic organisms, because mixed

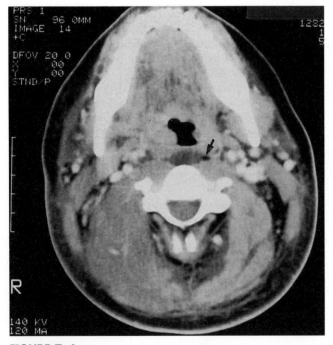

FIGURE 7–6
Computed tomography of a retropharyngeal abscess. (From Gidley PW, Steirnberg CM. Deep neck space infections. In Johnson JT, Yu VL [eds.]: *Infectious Diseases and Antimicrobial Therapy of the Ears, Nose, and Throat*, Philadelphia: WB Saunders, 1997.)

infections are the rule. The most common organisms include *Streptococcus, Staphylococcus, Bacteroides, Fusobacterium,* and *Peptostreptococcus.*

Patients with airway impairment, obvious large collections of pus, or those whose condition does not respond promptly to antibiotic therapy should be taken to the operating room, for incision and drainage under general anesthesia. Intubation must be meticulous, to avoid rupture of the abscess. The vast majority of retropharyngeal abscesses should be drained transorally. However, very large abscesses may require external drainage, particularly if infection has spread to the parapharyngeal space.

When to Refer

Patients with signs and symptoms of retropharyngeal abscess should be evaluated by an otolaryngologist or head and neck surgeon.

KEY POINTS

— Retropharyngeal abscess is most common in infants and young children.

— Do not palpate posterior pharyngeal swelling, as this may cause rupture of the abscess.

— With early diagnosis and treatment, some abscesses can be managed with intravenous antibiotics alone.

— Incision and drainage is usually required.

Suggested Readings

Brook I. Microbiology of retropharyngeal abscesses in children. *Am J Dis Child* 141:202–204, 1987.
Johnson J. Abscesses and deep space infections of the head and neck. *Infect Dis Clin North Am* 6:705–717, 1992.
Thompson J, Cohen SR, Reddix P. Retropharyngeal abscess in children: A retrospective and historical analysis. *Laryngoscope* 98:589–592, 1992.

Ludwig's Angina

Ludwig's angina is one of the most dangerous infections in the head and neck. It is a rapidly spreading, gangrenous, and putrid infection of the submaxillary space that can result in fatal airway obstruction. Inferior expansion is prevented by the strong deep cervical fascia, and therefore the massive swelling pushes the tongue and floor of mouth upward and backward, obstructing the oropharynx. This condition most often results from a dental infection, but it may also be caused by a mandible fracture or a submandibular gland infection.

Diagnosis

The diagnosis is readily apparent on the basis of characteristic physical signs: drooling, trismus, pain and swelling of the neck and floor of mouth, with woody edema and a foul smell. The tongue appears to be enlarged because it is pushed upward and backward into the mouth. Radiographs are rarely indicated, unless needed to rule out spread of infection to contiguous spaces.

Natural History

Untreated, the infection usually results in fatal airway obstruction within hours.

Treatment

The primary objective is to secure the airway. Orotracheal intubation is extremely difficult and inadvisable because trismus and brawny edema impair access to the larynx. Blind nasotracheal intubation is also dangerous. Fiberoptic intubation may be attempted in early cases, before swelling has progressed to a critical state of obstruction, but this requires an experienced and skilled clinician and a stable and cooperative patient. The safest means of securing airway patency is to perform a tracheotomy under local anesthesia.

Intravenous antibiotics are sometimes sufficient treatment for the infection, but surgical drainage is generally recommended. However, the infection generates little or no pus, and therefore incision does not significantly decompress the process. Thus, resolution of the airway compromise requires several days. As in most abscesses originating from the mouth or pharynx, multiple organisms are involved, including anaerobic species. Therefore, broad-spectrum antibiotic coverage is needed.

When to Refer

Because Ludwig's angina is such a rapidly progressive and frequently fatal illness, no time should be wasted in getting such a patient to an emergency facility, where airway patency can be established as soon as possible.

Parapharyngeal Abscess

Parapharyngeal abscess is the most common deep neck infection in adults. The parapharyngeal space is cone-shaped, widest near the base of the skull and tapering to its apex at the hyoid bone. It contains the important structures encased within the carotid sheath. Parapharyngeal abscess may result from a variety of sources, including the tonsils, adenoids, teeth, parotid gland, or sinuses. Intravenous drug use is also an increasingly common cause. An untreated mandible fracture may present with a parapharyngeal infection.

Patients present with fever, neck pain, dysphagia, and unilateral swelling and induration between the mandible and hyoid bone.

Diagnosis

The diagnosis is often obvious at presentation, owing to characteristic signs and symptoms of neck pain and fullness, which is maximal inferior and posterior to the angle of the mandible. However, because the abscess is located deeply in the neck, fluctuance is not often palpable. Therefore, it is usually not possible to differentiate cellulitis and abscess on the basis of findings on the physical examination. Computed tomography is usually required to identify and localize collections of pus and to determine whether surgical drainage is required (Fig. 7–7). Every effort should be made to identify and treat the source of the infection. This includes careful inspection of the teeth and gums.

Natural History

Complications of parapharyngeal abscess include internal jugular thrombosis, generalized sepsis, carotid hemorrhage, or spread of infection to adjacent spaces or the mediastinum. Significant airway compromise is not frequent; however, it may occur rapidly.

Treatment

Cellulitis and small abscesses may be amenable to medical management with broad-spectrum intravenous antibiotics. However, surgical drainage is always the safest option when there is a significant collection of pus. A parapharyngeal abscess should *never* be drained transorally, as this carries a high risk of injury to cranial nerves or to the carotid artery or the jugular vein. Further, an intraoral incision does not provide adequate drainage. Orotracheal intubation can be difficult, owing to trismus and pharyngeal distortion and the risk of rup-

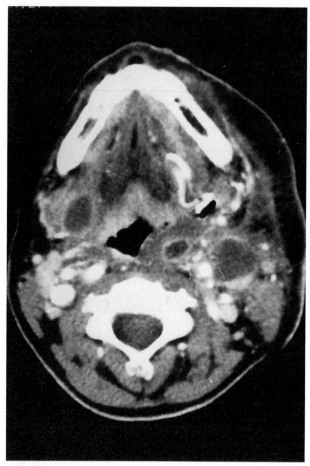

FIGURE 7–7
Computed tomography of a parapharyngeal abscess.

turing the abscess. Awake fiberoptic intubation is safer for establishing airway patency in difficult cases, but it requires experience and skill. Awake tracheotomy is always the safest option when the airway is in doubt.

KEY POINTS

— Parapharyngeal abscesses are rarely fluctuant to palpation.

— Computed tomography is required to detect abcesses that must be surgically drained.

— The source of the infection must be sought and treated.

— Most parapharyngeal abscesses result from dental infections.

Suggested Readings

Holt R, McManus K, Newman RK, Potter JL, Tinsley PP. Computed tomography in the diagnosis of deep neck infections. *Arch Otolaryngol Head Neck Surg* 108:693, 1982.

Myers EM, Kirkland LS, Mickey R. The head and neck sequelae of cervical intravenous drug abuse. *Laryngoscope* 98:213, 1988.

Gastroesophageal Reflux Pharyngitis

Gastroesophageal reflux pharyngitis is probably the most common cause of chronic sore throat in the adult population, but there are no reliable data on incidence and prevalence. Gastroesophageal reflux classically presents with such symptoms as heartburn, belching, and water brash but is frequently asymptomatic. Acid reflux alone rarely results in chronic pharyngitis. Generally, mucosal trauma is involved as a cofactor. This may result from an URI, voice abuse, coughing, or abrasion by a sharp ingested object, such as popcorn or a potato chip. Chronic gastroesophageal reflux irritates and delays healing of such minor injuries, resulting in chronic pain. Most often, reflux is intermittent rather than continual, but a single episode of reflux can produce symptoms lasting for days.

Patients with chronic gastroesophageal reflux pharyngitis present with throat pain that persists or recurs over several weeks. It is typically the worst in the morning. Patients may or may not relate symptoms of heartburn or belching but usually note a foul taste in the mouth on arising in the mornings. Pharyngeal swelling is usually perceived as postnasal drip or "something in the throat." Frequent efforts to clear the throat produce more local trauma, exacerbating the problem.

Diagnosis

Findings on physical examination of the mouth and oropharynx are usually unremarkable. Mirror examination or flexible nasopharyngoscopy may reveal a cherry-red inflammation of the hypopharynx or posterior glottis. Pooling of mucus or strands of mucus between the vocal folds are also significant signs. However, when symptoms result from inflammation in the tongue base, pyriform fossae, or upper cervical esophagus, physical signs may be subtle or invisible.

Barium swallow is useful when it demonstrates gastroesophageal reflux or a sliding hiatal hernia. However, because reflux is characteristically intermittent, false negatives are frequent, particularly in patients with nocturnal reflux. Barium swallow is also important in patients with complaints of dysphagia to evaluate the swallowing mechanism and to rule out aspiration.

Twenty-four-hour pH monitoring of the distal esophagus is generally regarded as the gold standard for diagnosis of gastroesophageal reflux resulting in esophagitis. However, its role in the management of reflux laryngitis or pharyngitis is unclear. Normative data on proximal esophageal pH is lacking. Although normal subjects frequently have occasional reflux into the distal esophagus, some authors feel that any episode of acid reaching the pharynx is abnormal. Moreover, because reflux episodes are usually intermittent, a 24-hour period of monitoring could be an inadequate sample.

The most cost-effective diagnostic test is an empiric trial of acid suppression. Relief from acid reflux does not result in instantaneous relief of symptoms; the damaged mucosa must heal. Therefore, trial therapy should be continued for at least 1 month, or even 2 months.

Flexible esophagoscopy may be indicated, particularly in patients with significant dysphagia, to document esophagitis and to detect possible strictures or webs.

Natural History

Chronic reflux pharyngitis may persist for months or years. Some patients experience relapsing and remitting symptoms. Repeat episodes may be precipitated by local trauma, such as coughing, ingestion of food with rough edges, or difficulty in swallowing large medication tablets. Increases in acid production, as in response to stress, has also been implicated. In some patients, a granulomatous mass forms in the larynx over the cartilage in the posterior vocal cord. Long-standing gastroesophageal reflux may play a role in the pathogenesis of laryngeal cancer. Acid reflux has been also implicated in the pathogenesis of chronic sinusitis and subglottic stenosis. Chronic reflux can also amplify symptoms in patients with asthma, owing to aspiration of reflux acid or to bronchospasm in response to esophageal irritation.

Chronic pharyngitis is often associated with chronic esophagitis, and both of these conditions can be complicated by overgrowth of *Candida*.

Treatment

Treatment of reflux pharyngitis is quite similar to management of reflux esophagitis, including medication to suppress acid secretion and enhance gastric emptying, diet modification, and elevation of the head of the bed at night.

In patients with mild to moderate symptoms, therapy with H_2 blockers may be adequate. However, in patients with significant symptoms or with a visible lesion on the larynx, H_2 blockers are unlikely to be successful and treatment with a proton pump inhibitor is indicated. Gastric emptying may be enhanced by a motility agent, such as metoclopramide. Small, frequent meals with no food or drink before retiring will decrease the volume of gastric material available for reflux.

Reflux pharyngitis does not resolve quickly. Often more month is required for resolution of symptoms, although physical of reflux generally begin to improve within 3–4 months. Treatm should be continued for at least 1 month after symptoms resolve, a minimum of 2 months, to allow for complete healing. Maintenance therapy with an H_2 blocker is recommended. In some patients, symptoms recur after discontinuation of the proton pump inhibitor and chronic therapy is required.

When to Refer

If a patient's sore throat persists beyond 2 months despite adequate reflux management, direct laryngoscopy and esophagoscopy are generally indicated to rule out other problems, such as an occult malignancy or esophageal candidiasis. If endoscopic findings are negative, gastroenterology consultation and 24-hour pH monitoring are indicated. Patients with significant recalcitrant pharyngitis may require fundoplication.

KEY POINTS

— Gastroesophageal reflux is an extremely common cause of chronic pharyngitis.

— Diagnosis is most effectively established by a therapeutic trial of acid suppression.

— When medical therapy fails, endoscopy is required to rule out other lesions and potential malignancy.

— In recalcitrant pharyngitis, consideration should be given to fundoplication.

Suggested Readings

Ahuja V, Yencha MW, Lasseu LF. Head and neck manifestations of gastroesophageal reflux disease. *Am Fam Physician* 60:873–880, 885–886, 1999.

Other Inflammatory Disorders of the Throat

Angioedema

Angioedema is focal swelling of the face, oral cavity, oropharynx, and/or larynx due to venule and capillary dilation and increased vascular permeability. This can lead to life-threatening airway obstruction. Angioedema may be hereditary, owing to a deficiency of C1 exercise inhibitor, but it may also result from allergy to drugs or insect bites

ıs. An increasingly common cause of angioedema
ıtensin-converting enzyme (ACE) inhibitors, used
hypertension.

ıte episodes should include epinephrine, cortico-
ımines, although these are less effective in man-
.ιor reactions. Recurrent attacks of hereditary angi-
. ɔan be diminished by chronic administration of danazol.

Benign Mucosal Ulceration

Various inflammatory processes can result in ulceration of the oral
or pharyngeal mucosa. The most common such problem is minor
recurrent aphthous stomatitis, and idiopathic disorders. Minor ulcers
are less than 1 cm in diameter, usually last 7–10 days, and heal
without scarring. Major aphthous stomatitis is much less common
and produces larger ulcers, lasting weeks to months and eventually
healing with significant scarring. Major aphthous ulcers usually occur
in the mouth but may involve the pharynx or larynx. Numerous
remedies have been used, including topical steroids and systemic
anti-inflammatory agents, none with proven efficacy.

Lupus, pemphigus, pemphigoid, and lichen planus can all produce
lesions and ulcers in the mouth. Diagnosis is established by biopsy.

8

SALIVARY GLAND DISORDERS

I N T R O D U C T I O N

There are thousands of salivary glands in the head and neck region. However, salivary disorders are predominantly manifested in two pairs of major salivary glands: the parotid and submandibular glands. These glands are characterized by complex duct systems. Most inflammatory disorders involve some degree of obstruction of the ducts, resulting in swelling. Tumors present as expanding masses. It is therefore not surprising that the most common presenting sign of salivary gland disease, regardless of pathology, is enlargement of the infected gland. Pain, resulting from infection, pressure within obstructed ducts, or local extravasation of saliva, is more common in non-neoplastic disease. Tumors tend to be more slowly growing. Facial nerve weakness is an ominous sign, generally associated with malignancy.

Acute Viral Parotitis

The most common viral infection of the parotid gland is mumps. This is predominantly a disease of childhood. Peak incidence is from between the ages of 4 and 6 years. It is caused by a highly contagious systemic myxovirus, with an incubation period of 14–21 days. The virus is spread by airborne droplets if saliva and nasal secretions, as well as urine. The incidence of mumps infection has reduced by more than 90% since 1977, when routine vaccination was introduced.

Other viral causes of salivary gland infection include cytomegalovirus (CMV) and coxsackievirus.

Presentation

There is commonly a prodrome of fever, malaise, and headache. Then one parotid gland swells. In most cases, the second gland also becomes involved. Ingestion of food, particularly sour-tasting food, increases the pain. Other possible signs and symptoms include trismus, eyelid swelling, and edema of the external auditory canal.

Diagnosis

Diagnosis of mumps is usually obvious on the basis of physical findings of painful parotid swelling and systemic malaise. The patient is often aware of recent exposure to the disease and clearly recognizes the symptoms. Stensen's duct orifice is usually erythemetous. Saliva remains clear during mumps, in contrast to the purulent saliva that is characteristic of bacterial infection. Definitive diagnosis can be established by detection of viral antigens in the blood and urine. Other positive blood test results include leukopenia and increased serum amylase.

Cytomegalovirus infection produces symptoms similar to those of infectious mononucleosis, such as fever, hepatosplenomegaly, jaundice, lymphadenopathy, leukopenia, and thrombocytopenia. Coxsackievirus infection is frequently associated with gingivitis and pharyngitis.

Natural History

Mumps is most frequently a benign disorder that resolves within 1 week or so. Other salivary glands may become inflamed. Involvement of other organs may result in complications, such as deafness, encephalitis, orchitis, and/or pancreatitis. Menigitis is the most common complication. After puberty, mumps orchitis carries a 30% risk of sterility. Rarely, ovaries may become involved. Mumps infection may result in chronic obstructive sialadenitis, a condition with significant long-term morbidity.

The course of parotid CMV infection is very similar to that of infectious mononucleosis. Occasionally CMV may cause hepatitis, myocarditis, polyradiculitis, or Guillain-Barré syndrome.

Treatment

There is currently no specifically effective treatment for viral infection of salivary glands. Clinical management is supportive. Some have recommended gammaglobulin for men with mumps, to prevent orchitis.

The mainstay of management of mumps is prevention, not treatment. All children older than 12 months should receive a measles-mumps-rubella vaccine, with a second dose at entry into school. Any older person considered susceptible to mumps should also be immunized. Anyone born before 1957 is almost assuredly immune to mumps, having had overt or subclinical infection. Those born later should be assumed to be susceptible unless there is documentation of immunization, diagnosed mumps, or serologic evidence of immunity.

When to Refer

Uncomplicated viral parotitis resolves without specific therapy. Referral may be indicated for management of specific complications.

KEY POINTS

— In viral parotitis, saliva is clear, not purulent.

— Mumps is generally a benign disease but may be complicated by deafness, pancreatitis, encephalitis, or orchitis.

— In men, sterility is a potential complication of mumps.

— Mumps infection may cause chronic recurrent sialadenitis.

Acute Bacterial Sialadenitis

In healthy salivary glands, salivary flow continually flushes out the ducts. Acute bacterial infection of the parotid or submandibular gland results from stasis of saliva, with reflux of oral bacteria. Stasis may be the result of duct obstruction (due to stricture, stones, trauma, or oral infection) or reduced salivary secretion (due to dehydration, anticholinergic medication, or lack of oral intake). Salivary flow is commonly reduced in patients who have just undergone surgery, owing to dehydration and lack of eating, and it is therefore not surprising that approximately one third of cases of parotitis occur after surgery. Bilateral involvement is common in postoperative parotitis. Dehydration rarely causes infection of the submandibular glands, presumably because submandibular secretions are predominantly mucous in nature rather than proteolytic. Other risk factors for bacterial sialadenitis include cystic fibrosis, because of extremely viscous saliva, and acquired immunodeficiency syndrome (AIDS). Parotitis is most commonly due to *Staphylococcus,* whereas oral flora predominate in the submandibular gland.

Presentation

Presenting signs and symptoms include pain, tenderness, and swelling of affected glands; a metallic taste in the mouth; and increased pain on eating. Some patients, particularly those who are elderly or debilitated, have systemic symptoms of fever, chills, and malaise.

Diagnosis

Diagnosis is based on the physical finding of a painful, swollen gland. The orifice of the duct is red and swollen, and massage of the gland often expresses pus. This should be cultured prior to initiation of antibiotic therapy. There may be regional adenopathy. Adjunctive studies or laboratory tests are not generally indicated. However, computed tomography (CT) or ultrasound may be useful to detect abscess formation. Sialography is not advisable during an acute infection.

Natural History

Increased pressure in the parotid duct system leads to leakage of fluid into surrounding tissue, with autodigestion of parenchyma and microabscess formation. This may progress to frank abscess cavity formation, manifested by progressive edema and induration of the overlying tissues. Fluctuance is not often palpable on physical examination, owing to the dense capsule of this gland. If antibiotic therapy does not result in improvement within a few days or if disease progresses despite adequate treatment, the possibility of abscess formation should be assessed by CT or ultrasound.

Abscess formation is rare in the submandibular gland, presumably because of the predominance of mucus over proteolytic secretion. Intraductal scarring may develop in either gland as the result of the infection, predisposing the patient to recurrent or chronic infection.

Treatment

Antibiotics should be prescribed to cover the most common organisms, *Staphylococcus* in the parotid and oral flora in the submandibular gland. As stasis is a major factor in the pathogenesis of the infection, treatment includes measures to promote drainage, such as hydration, gentle massage, local application of heat, and the use of sialogogues to stimulate secretion. Some have recommended the use of trypsin inactivator factor to limit parenchymal damage.

If saliva does not flow freely, the duct orifice should be gently dilated, using lacrimal probes. If this is not successful in establishing salivary flow, then obstruction of the duct, by stricture or a stone, should be suspected. Open surgical drainage is indicated for known abscesses. If the infection does not respond to medical treatment within 48 hours, an abscess should be presumed.

When to Refer

Otolaryngologic consultation is indicated when infection is due to obstruction or when abscess is suspected.

KEY POINTS

— Acute bacterial sialadenitis results from stasis due to dehydration or obstruction.

— Treatment includes antibiotics and measures to reestablish salivary drainage.

— Abscessed glands remain firm and do not fluctuate.

— Surgical drainage is required if medical management fails.

— Acute sialadenitis may lead to chronic and recurrent sialadenitis.

Suggested Reading

Brook I. Diagnosis and management of parotitis. *Arch Otolaryngol Head Neck Surg* 118:469–471, 1992.

Chronic Recurrent Sialadenitis

Any infection of the parotid or submandibular gland can result in duct stricture, sialactasis, parenchymal damage, or chronic inflammation. Such changes impair salivary drainage, predisposing the patient to recurrent infections. Stagnant saliva is easily inoculated by reflux of oral bacteria.

Presentation

Signs and symptoms of each recurrent infection are quite similar to those of an isolated acute infection, with pain and swelling of the involved gland. Between acute infections, patients may have symptoms of partial duct obstruction, with painful swelling of the gland during meals.

Diagnosis

In this disorder, the history is so characteristic that patient interview is sufficient to support a presumptive diagnosis, even if the patient is between acute episodes and completely asymptomatic at the time of initial examination. Other considerations in the differential diagnosis include salivary stones and autoimmune sialadenitis (Sjögren's syndrome); however, the initial clinical management of the quiescent phase of all three disorders is identical: supportive and palliative measures only.

The intraoral orifice of the duct should be examined for inflammation and the gland should be massaged as the punctum is observed, to determine the nature of salivary drainage. But when a patient with a history of recurrent sialadenitis presents with an acutely swollen gland, bacterial infection should always be presumed, even when no pus can be expressed. Drainage of purulent saliva is clear evidence of an acute infection. If no saliva can be expressed, then the gland is totally obstructed, by scarring or calculi; if some clear saliva can be expressed, partial obstruction is possible. In either case, one cannot exclude the possibility of a loculated bacterial infection.

Sialography should be performed, after resolution of acute infection, to detect the presence of any stones (Figs. 8–1 and 8–2). Sialography is also helpful in documenting the severity of disease. Commonly, the duct system has a "pruned tree" pattern, with stretched and tapered ducts, a decrease in duct number, and absence of acinar filling. Focal areas of the duct may be dilated, appearing as a string of sausage links.

Natural History

Management of this disorder is frustrating. It is chronic and progressive. Although acute flare-ups can be treated, each acute episode contributes to the severity of the problem. With progression, acute infections become more frequent. Between infections, patients develop symptoms of decreasing salivary function, with a dry mouth or prob-

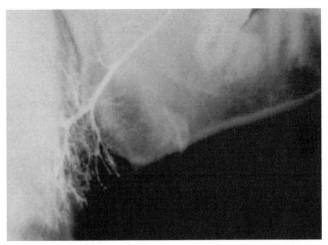

FIGURE 8-1
A normal parotid sialogram. (From Blitzer CE, Lawson W, Reino A. Sialadenitis. In Johnson JT, Yu VL [eds.]: *Infectious Diseases and Antimicrobial Therapy of the Ears, Nose, and Throat*, Philadelphia: WB Saunders, 1997.)

lems with partial obstruction, so that the gland swells painfully during meals. There is little that the physician can do to directly alter the progression of disease.

Treatment

The management of each recurrent infection is quite similar to that of an isolated bacterial infection. Antibiotics should be prescribed to

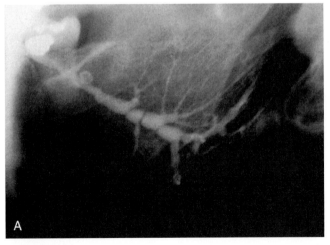

FIGURE 8-2
Sialogram of patient with chronic sialadenitis showing sausage link–like patterns and massive duct dilation. (From Blitzer CE, Lawson W, Reino A. Sialadenitis. In Johnson JT, Yu VL [eds.]: *Infectious Diseases and Antimicrobial Therapy of the Ears, Nose, and Throat*, Philadelphia: WB Saunders, 1997.)

cover the most commonly identified pathogens, including *Staphylococcus, Haemophilus,* and *Streptococcus.* As in any recurrent infectious process, the development of antibiotic resistance is a concern. If purulence can be expressed from the gland orifice, a specimen should be sent for culture and sensitivity and antibiotics should be adjusted appropriately. Other treatment measures include gland massage, hydration, and local application of heat.

Patients should be counseled regarding the chronic and progressive nature of this disease and instructed in measures to decrease the incidence of recurrent infection. It is important to maintain adequate fluid intake, as dehydration leads to decreased salivation and stasis. The use of sialogogues, such as lemon drops, assist in maintaining salivary flow. Mucolytic agents, such as guaifenesin, should be used to decrease the viscosity of saliva. Frequent gland massage aids in emptying ectatic ducts. Patients should avoid the use of any medication that decreases salivation, such as most antihistamine preparations.

When medical management fails to control the progression of disease and the morbidity of obstructive symptoms and recurrent infections outweighs the risks of surgery, then complete excision of the gland is indicated. Surgical excision of a chronically infected submandibular gland is a fairly simple procedure; however, total parotidectomy in a patient with chronic parotitis is technically challenging. Fibrosis and bleeding make dissection of the facial nerve more difficult, increasing the risk of injury.

When to Refer

Chronic sialadenitis is a progressive disease that significantly affects the patient's quality of life and may ultimately require surgery. It is therefore appropriate for an otolaryngologist to be involved in management of chronic disease.

KEY POINTS

— Recurrent and chronic sialadenitis results from impaired salivary drainage.

— No medical therapy is effective.

— Conservative measures to improve salivary flow can retard or halt disease progression.

— Definitive treatment is surgical excision of the gland.

Suggested Reading

O'Brien CJ, Murrant HJ. Surgical management of chronic parotitis. *Head Neck* 13:445–449, 1993.

Sjögren's Syndrome

Sjögren's syndrome is a collagen vascular disorder consisting of kera- toconjunctivitis sicca and xerostomia. In primary Sjögren's sydrome, involvement is limited to the lacrimal and salivary glands. Secondary Sjögren's syndrome includes systemic autoimmune disease, such as systemic lupus erythematosus (SLE), scleroderma, polymyositis, or peirarteritis nodosa. Other systemic diseases occasionally associated with Sjögren's syndrome include macrocytic anemia, pancreatitis, diabetes mellitus, Hashimoto's thyroiditis, and lymphoma.

Presentation

Age of onset of Sjögren's syndrome is typically between 50 and 60 years. Patients present with complaints referrable to salivary and/ or lacrimal gland involvement. Decreased salivation may be mani- fested by symptoms of oral dryness, difficulty swallowing, halitosis, or chronic sore throat. Ocular symptoms include burning, a sensation of having a foreign body, and light sensitivity. Patients often note facial swelling due to parotid gland enlargement. In secondary Sjö- gren's syndrome, patients also have signs and symptoms of associated rheumatoid disease, such as arthritis, scleroderma, SLE, or polymyo- sitis.

Diagnosis

Physical examination usually reveals symmetric nontender swelling of the parotid glands (Fig. 8–3). Less commonly, the submandibular glands are also involved.

There are no available tests for reliably quantifying salivary production. Lacrimal function may be assessed by a simple office test, the Schirmer's test. A short, narrow strip of filter paper (approximately 5×20 mm) is used for this test. A transverse fold is created 3–4 mm from one end, and this end is placed just under the lower eyelid. The other end is allowed to hang freely. Tears are absorbed by and conducted along the paper. With normal lacrimal function, the paper should become wet for at least 6 mm from the eyelid.

The diagnosis is confirmed by biopsy of the lower lip, for histologic examination of minor salivary glands. Pathologic changes include acinar atrophy and lymphocytic infiltration. There is an increase in immunoglobulin (Ig) G containing plasma cells. Antibodies against cytoplasmic antigens of salivary duct epithelium (anti-Sjögren's anti- bodies A and B) can be detected in the serum. Although technically difficult, it is sometimes possible to collect saliva for chemical testing. Characteristic changes in saliva from Sjögren's patients include in- creased sodium, IgA, IgG, lactoferrin, and albumin and decreased

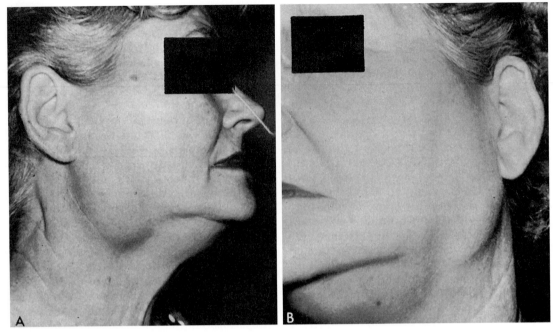

FIGURE 8-3

Sixty-year-old woman had bilateral benign lymphoepithelial disease of both parotid glands for a number of years. Cavitary sialectasis was present, according to sialographic studies. Infection was evident on numerous occasions. Because of persistent enlargement and infection, bilateral parotidectomies with preservation of both facial nerves were performed in staged operations. The patient has remained well without disability. (From Work WP, Hecht DW. Inflammatory diseases of the major salivary glands. In Paparella MM, Shumrick DA [eds.]: *Otolaryngology,* vol. 3, Philadelphia: WB Saunders, 1980.)

phosphate. Sialography is usually unnecessary for diagnosis and does not provide information that would distinguish Sjögren's from chronic sialadenitis.

Natural History

Sjögren's syndrome is a chronic condition that does not resolve spontaneously. There is a potential for development of lymphatic malignancy.

Treatment

There is no really effective treatment for Sjögren's syndrome. Supportive measures include the use of artificial tears and saliva. Infections must be treated with the usual measures for sialadenitis, including antibiotics, hydration, gentle massage, and sialogogues.

When to Refer

If conservative measures do not control chronic and recurrent parotid infection, then total parotidectomy may be indicated. If a mass develops, malignancy should be suspected. Such patients should be referred for consideration of possible surgical management.

KEY POINTS

— Sjögren's syndrome should be suspected in patients with symptoms of dry mouth and eyes, particularly when accompanied by parotid gland enlargement and/or signs or rheumatic disease.

— Diagnosis is established by histologic evaluation of minor salivary glands in a lip biopsy.

— Only supportive treatment is available.

— Surgical excision should be considered for uncontrolled infections or suspected development of malignancy.

Salivary Stones (Sialolithiasis)

Stones are much more common in the submandibular gland than in the parotid. Submandibular secretions are more viscous and thus more likely to form concretions. Stones are formed by calcification around a nidus of inspissated mucus or ductal debris. A common location is just inside the duct orifice. In the submandibular gland, another frequent site is that portion of the duct which passes over the mylohyoid muscle. Multiple stones may occur. Cystic fibrosis, which causes increased viscosity of all exocrine secretions, is associated with an increased incidence of salivary stones.

Presentation

The sequellae of salivary stones derive solely from the obstruction they cause. Partial obstruction impairs flow during peak secretory flow, during eating. This causes pain and swelling of the gland with eating, which gradually subside after the meal. The gland generally returns to normal as the saliva gradually drains out; however, partial obstruction can lead to acute bacterial sialadenitis. Total obstruction of the duct leads to chronic enlargement, frequently with bacterial infection (Fig. 8–4).

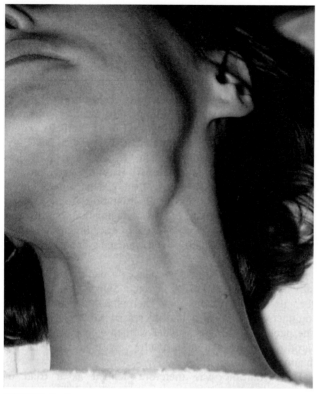

FIGURE 8-4
Patient with large calculus and obstruction of the left submandibular gland. (From Blitzer CE, Lawson W, Reino A. Sialadenitis. In Johnson JT, Yu VL [eds.]: *Infectious Diseases and Antimicrobial Therapy of the Ears, Nose, and Throat,* Philadelphia: WB Saunders, 1997.)

Diagnosis

A history of chronic or recurrent rapid and painful gland enlargement associated with eating is highly suggestive of a salivary stone. Submandibular stones may sometimes be detected by bimanual palpation of the floor of the mouth, or may even be visible as submucosal swelling. The duct orifice should be probed with lacrimal probes to rule out stricture, and possibly to release a stone at that location.

Submental occlusal dental radiographs are often helpful in demonstrating submandibular salivary calculi; however, 20% of submandibular stones are radiolucent. Plain radiography is less helpful in the parotid gland, where 40% of stones are radiolucent. Posteroanterior and lateral skull views should be used to detect parotid stones. If stones are suspected but not demonstrated on plain films, then contrast sialography may be used. A cannula is introduced into the duct orifice and contrast material is injected. Strictures, calculi, and ductal ectasia are easily demonstrated by this technique. Postinjection films demonstrate the degree of filling and emptying. Sialography is contraindicated in patients with a history of allergy to contrast material and should not be performed during an acute infection.

Treatment

If possible, the stones should be removed transorally, by dilating the duct and massaging the gland. If necessary, the duct wall may be incised over an indwelling probe to release the stone. Because of the risk of nerve or vessel damage, the duct should not be incised more than 2 cm from the punctum. Successful removal of the stone is heralded by a sudden outflow of saliva or pus. If the intraoral approach fails, then surgical excision of the gland is indicated.

KEY POINTS

— Stones are common in the submandibular duct but uncommon in the parotid.

— Submandibular stones may be palpable in the floor of the mouth.

— Most submandibular gland calculi are radiopaque, whereas 60% of parotid stones are radiolucent.

— Intraoral removal is preferrable, but complete excision of the gland may ultimately be required.

Suggested Reading

Williams MF. Sialolithiasis. *Otolaryngol Clin North Am* 32:819–834, 1999.

Ranula

A retention cyst in the anterior floor of the mouth is called a ranula. This term is derived from the Latin word for frog because the appearance of this cyst has been likened to that of a frog's belly. A ranula represents cystic dilation of either a sublingual gland or the submandibular duct. It may occur as a developmental anomaly or may be acquired. It is thin walled and filled with mucus. A simple ranula is a true cyst, whereas a "plunging" ranula is a pseudocyst formed by extravasation of saliva into local soft tissues.

Presentation

A ranula presents as a smooth, soft swelling in the anterior floor of the mouth. It may have a bluish tinge. Patients complain of fullness and sometimes pain in that location.

Natural History

The usual clinical course is gradual enlargement of the cyst. Significant fluctuation is size is quite common, owing to periodic rupture and decompression with subsequent reaccumulation of saliva. The danger of ranulas is that rupture may occur on the deep surface rather than into the mouth. Such rupture leads to extravasation of saliva into the tissues of the floor of the mouth and formation of a pseudocyst that gradually dissects inferiorly. This is called a "plunging" ranula. Occasionally, a plunging ranula extends ominously into the mediastinum. The worst complication would be mediastinitis. It is important to recognize and treat this innocent-appearing lesion early rather than late.

Treatment

A ranula must be surgically treated, either by excision or marsupialization. Excision is theoretically preferrable but in practice often results in recurrence because the thin, delicate cyst wall frequently ruptures during surgery. In fact, previous rupture is common, resulting in defects in the cyst wall and associated pseudocyst formation. It is not possible to completely excise a pseudocyst. Thus, the most effective treatment is usually marsupialization. A portion of the intraoral mucosa is removed en bloc with an underlying portion of the cyst wall. The intraoral mucosa is then sutured to the adjacent cyst wall. Even with appropriate surgery, recurrence is common. It is important to persevere with revision surgery until definitive treatment is achieved, owing to the potential complications of an untreated ranula.

When to Refer

Any persisting cystic lesion in the mouth should be referred for possible surgical management.

KEY POINTS

— A smooth, soft submucosal mass in the floor of the mouth is most likely a ranula.

— A ranula may be a well-circumscribed cyst or a "plunging" pseudocyst, possibly extending into the mediastinum.

— Surgical marsupialization is usually the treatment of choice.

Suggested Reading

Davison MJ, Morton MP. Plunging ranula: clinical observation. *Head Neck* 20:63–68, 1998.

Salivary Gland Tumors

A lump in a salivary gland should be assumed to be a tumor until proven otherwise, because of the importance of early treatment for salivary tumors. Other causes of salivary masses include infection, postinflammatory scarring, focal duct obstruction, or, in the parotid gland, an enlarged lymph node.

Parotid lymph nodes drain the scalp and auricular area and may be enlarged because of infection of these areas. Cat-scratch lymphadenitis may present as a parotid mass, especially in children. An enlarged node may also represent a lymphatic tumor or a metastasis from a cutaneous tumor, such as squamous carcinoma.

A variety of histologic types of tumors arise in salivary glands, both benign and malignant. In general, the smaller the salivary gland, the greater is the risk of malignancy. For example, tumors of the minor salivary glands are most likely to be adenoid cystic carcinoma, an insidious, slow-growing tumor with an extremely high mortality rate. On the other hand, the vast majority of parotid tumors are benign; 65% are one specific type—benign mixed tumor. In children, the most common noninflammatory mass is a hemangioma.

Presentation

A parotid tumor commonly presents as a painless, slowly growing mass on the side of the face. A submandibular gland tumor presents as diffuse enlargement just below the body of the mandible. Sometimes a patient with a salivary tumor notes facial asymmetry or feels a mass when washing. However, salivary gland masses are quite frequently detected incidentally on routine physical examination. Minor salivary gland tumors, which are rare, present as submucosal nodules or cysts in the mouth. Small cysts in the oral mucosa are nearly always benign mucoceles, but very occasionally they are malignant tumors.

Diagnosis

Evaluation of a salivary mass is similar to the workup of a neck mass. As in neck masses, an inflammatory cause is more common among children, whereas neoplasia is more common among adults. A history of previous salivary gland infection or stones increases the likelihood that the mass represents inflammation or scarring. Rapid growth and tenderness are signs of an active inflammatory process. Conversely, a slowly growing painless mass should be regarded as a tumor until proven otherwise.

Parotid gland masses typically present in the preauricular area, or just below the lobule. The scalp and skin of the head and neck should be carefully inspected for infection or lesions, with particular attention given to seeking potential carcinoma or melanoma. Intraoral evaluation may reveal displacement of the palate or tonsil by parapharyngeal extension of a deep-lobe parotid tumor. The neck should be carefully palpated for adenopathy.

Because submandibular gland tumors typically present as a firm enlargement of the entire gland rather than as a discrete mass, it is very difficult to differentiate between tumor and other causes of gland enlargement, such as lithiasis or postinflammatory scarring. As in patients with parotid masses, the neck should be carefully palpated for possible metastasis. The marginal mandibular branch of the facial nerve may be involved by submandibular malignancy; therefore, lower lip function should be carefully evaluated.

Plain films of the salivary glands are only useful when the presence of stones is suspected. Computed tomography is rarely necessary for submandibular gland disease but is often helpful for parotid masses, particularly when parapharyngeal extension is suspected.

Fine-needle aspiration (FNA) is an extremely valuable tool. This technique is described in Chapter 11. Cytologic examination of cells aspirated from the mass can usually distinguish between inflammatory and neoplastic process. Specific tumor histology can be identified with a high degree of accuracy. Occasionally FNA will obviate the need for surgery by identifying a treatable inflammatory process or a tumor that is unlikely to result in problems; however, the vast majority of salivary gland masses require excisional biopsy to simultaneously treat and confirm the diagnosis.

Natural History

The most common tumor of the parotid gland, the benign mixed tumor, does not metastasize or invade but does grow relentlessly and can reach a very large size. Occasionally, local compression can impair function of the facial nerve; however, the association of facial weakness with a parotid mass usually indicates malignancy. Malignant transformation does occur in benign mixed tumors.

The clinical behavior of malignant salivary gland tumors varies greatly, depending on the specific histologic type. For example, a low-grade mucoepidermoid tumor is not likely to recur or metastasize. At the other end of the spectrum, adenoid cystic carcinoma is a slowly growing but highly malignant tumor with a strong propensity for perineural invasion, local recurrance, and distant metastasis. Adenoid cystic carcinoma is nearly always fatal, but the disease course is prolonged, sometimes up to 20 years.

Treatment

Most noninflammatory salivary gland masses should be surgically excised. Occasionally, FNA will obviate the need for surgery. Warthin's tumor (cystadenoma lymphomatosum) is a slowly growing benign tumor that is most common in elderly men. If this tumor type is clearly demonstrated by cytology and the patient is over 60 years of age and not concerned by the appearance of the lump, then it is reasonable to defer surgery. The patient should be monitored with serial physical examinations, with an eye toward changes in consistency or acceleration of growth rate. In general, all other tumors should be removed, owing to the risk of facial nerve impairment by an expanding tumor or the possibility of malignant transformation.

The minimum surgical procedure for a parotid mass is superficial parotidectomy, removing that portion of the gland lateral to the facial nerve. If it is a deep-lobe tumor, then the minimum procedure is a total parotidectomy. To treat a submandibular mass, the entire gland should be excised. The excised specimen should be immediately examined histologically, using frozen section. When a malignant tumor is detected, some intraoperative decisions must be made. For some malignant tumors, concomitant neck dissection is indicated. Sometimes, the facial nerve must be sacrificed, as when the nerve is encased by tumor or adherent to it.

When to Refer

An otolaryngologist or other head and neck surgeon should evaluate all parotid gland masses and submandibular gland enlargement.

KEY POINTS

— A mass in the parotid gland should be regarded as a tumor until proven otherwise.

— Firm enlargement of the submandibular gland may represent a tumor or chronic obstruction.

— All suspected salivary tumors should be referred for possible surgical management.

— Fine-needle aspiration cytology is a valuable tool in the diagnosis of salivary gland masses.

— Benign mixed tumors of the parotid gland may undergo malignant degeneration.

— The minimal surgery for a salivary gland mass is superficial parotidectomy, and for submandibular gland enlargement, total excision.

— Malignant tumors may require neck dissection, radiotherapy, and/or sacrifice of the facial nerve.

Suggested Reading

Candel A, Gattuso P, Reddy V, Matz G, Castelli M. Is fine needle aspiration biopsy of salivary gland masses really necessary? *Ear Nose Throat J* 72:485–489, 1993.

Sadeghi A, Tran LM, Mark R, Sidrys J, Parlor RG. Minor salivary gland tumors of the head and neck: treatment strategies and prognosis. *Am J Clin Oncol* 16:3–8, 1993.

Less Common Parotid Gland Disorders

The parotid and lacrimal glands may become enlarged in patients with sarcoidosis (uveoparotid fever). Diagnosis is established by FNA or open biopsy. No effective treatment is available.

Parotid gland enlargement is frequently encountered in patients with AIDS. Such enlargement is most often due to benign cystic lesions, which can be managed conservatively by repetitive needle aspiration. Surgical excision is not indicated for benign cysts; however, B-cell lymphoma may arise in the parotid glands of these patients. Therefore, aspirated material should be carefully evaluated cytologically, because malignant tumors should be treated aggressively.

Salivary gland enlargement is reported to occur in approximately 30% of patients with bulemia. It is generally benign and resolves once the disease is controlled.

Fatty infiltration and hypertrophy of the parotid occurs in alchoholism and kwashiorkor. The parotid gland may become infected with tuberculosis, cat-scratch disease, or actinomyces. Occasionally, a branchial cleft cyst will present with parotid enlargement.

Suggested Reading

Rice DH. Salivary gland disorders: neoplastic and non-neoplastic. *Med Clin North Am* 83:197–218, xi, 1999.

9

VOICE DISORDERS

I N T R O D U C T I O N

Many different disease processes can impair the voice, and so it is not surprising that hoarseness is one of the most common symptoms encountered in clinical practice. Even minute lesions of the vocal fold can interfere with vibration. Neurologic disorders can also affect the voice, because speech is a complex function involving the precise and integrated activity of different organ systems. A brief review of the physiology of voice production will elucidate the various mechanisms of hoarseness.

The voice is produced by passive oscillation of the vocal folds, powered by exhaled air. This process, called phonation, will not occur unless several physical requirements are met:

- The glottis must be loosely closed, with light contact between the vocal folds. If closure is tight, high pressure will be required to force the vocal folds open and begin vibration; the voice will sound tight and strained. If

157

closure is too loose, there will be excess airflow and the voice will sound weak and breathy.

- There must be adequate airflow and pressure. Normal expiratory airflow is more than adequate for conversational speech, and so the voice is usually not impaired by mild to moderate pulmonary disease. However, impaired pulmonary function can reduce the capacity to use increased airflow to compensate for other vocal pathology.

- The mucosal cover of the vocal fold is normally separated from the underlying muscle by a layer of loose connective tissue. This microanatomic arrangement allows the mucosa to vibrate freely. Scar tissue or edema can impair vibration. Figure 9–1 is a diagram of the structure of a vocal fold, in coronal section.

- Mucus secretion is another important factor in vocal function. A mucous blanket lubricates the vocal fold to reduce shearing force. The mucus also maintains hydration. This is important because more pressure is required to generate sound when the vocal folds are dehydrated.

TABLE 9–1 • **REQUIREMENTS FOR NORMAL PHONATION**

Loosely approximated glottis
Adequate expiratory airflow and pressure
Supple, homogenous vocal fold mucosa
Appropriate mucus secretion
Control of vocal fold length and tension

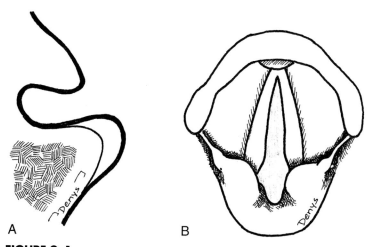

FIGURE 9–1
Diagram of normal vocal fold structure, **A,** coronal section, **B,** viewed from above.

> • Pitch is controlled by changes in length and tension of
> the vocal folds. Defects in motor control can produce
> vocal instability.

Acute Laryngitis

Virtually everyone has occasionally experienced hoarseness due to acute inflammation of the larynx. The most common causes include upper respiratory infection (URI), vocal abuse, and gastroesophageal reflux (Table 9–2). In many patients, more than one contributing factor can be identified. During an URI, laryngeal inflammation generally results from the trauma of coughing or from irritation from infected drainage—the infection does not usually involve the larynx itself. Both coughing and vocal abuse (shouting and loud talking) exert the vocal folds. This force is maximal on the posterior ends of the vocal folds, which are composed of cartilage covered by mucosa. The compression between the arytenoid cartilages can damage the mucosal cover. Gastroesophageal reflux contributes to posterior laryngeal injury because it primarily affects the mucosa

TABLE 9–2 • **COMMON CAUSES OF LARYNGITIS**

Upper respiratory infection
Voice abuse
Gastroesophageal reflux

near the esophageal inlet. Thus, in most cases of acute laryngitis, hoarseness is not due to inflammation of the vocal folds per se. Inflammation is maximal in the tissues of the posterior larynx, and this prevents the vocal folds from approximating adequately.

Presentation

Hoarseness is most often first noted on awakening in the morning. In other cases, the first sign of such inflammation is that increasing effort is required to speak. As the patient continues to speak, it becomes increasingly difficult to make a sound and the voice becomes raspy or breathy. With severe edema, the voice may be lost completely. Pain is variable. Dyspnea is not a symptom of common laryngitis, because the edema is not sufficient to compromise the airway. The primary problem is in fact the inability to close the larynx.

Diagnosis

The diagnosis of laryngitis is usually apparent from the history and the sound of the patient's voice. The cause of the laryngitis is also apparent from the history. Patients commonly recognize the connection between an URI and hoarseness. If the patient has been cheering loudly at a sporting event the night before, the vocal abuse can be identified as a factor. Gastroesophageal reflux may be implicated by a history of reflux symptoms, such as belching, heartburn, or water brash. Often the patient does not note any symptoms of reflux, because the esophagus is not inflamed or because reflux occurs during sleep. However, reflux should be strongly suspected if hoarseness occurs after a patient has gone to bed soon after a large meal or after drinking alcohol. A foul taste in the mouth on awakening is another sign of nocturnal reflux.

As mentioned previously, common laryngitis does not result in airway obstruction. Therefore, if a patient complains of dyspnea or stridor is noted, then another diagnosis should be strongly considered.

Physical examination should include inspection of the nose, mouth, and oropharynx, to seek signs of URI, sinusitis, or tonsillitis.

Examination of the larynx should primarily focus on ruling out other causes of hoarseness. It is important to confirm that the vocal folds move normally and that there are no lesions on the vocal folds. The physical findings of laryngitis may be subtle. Sometimes the only observable evidence of posterior laryngeal edema is incomplete glottic closure (Fig. 9–2). With experience, it becomes easier to recognize the signs of posterior laryngitis, such as erythema or ulceration of the vocal processes, mucus stranding between the vocal folds, thickening of posterior glottic tissue, and a violaeceous shelf beneath the vocal folds.

Natural History

Acute laryngitis generally resolves spontaneously over 1–2 weeks. However, if conditions that irritate the larynx persist, hoarseness may not resolve and chronic laryngitis may develop. It is important to note that laryngitis precipitated by one factor may be prolonged by other factors. For example, it is not uncommon for a patient with acute laryngitis from an URI to develop chronic laryngitis because of preexisting gastroesophageal reflux or poor vocal habits.

Treatment

Treatment of acute laryngitis should be symptom based and supportive, allowing for spontaneous resolution. If hoarseness is severe, vocal use should be restricted. Absolute silence is very difficult to maintain and is not necessary. However, patients should refrain from

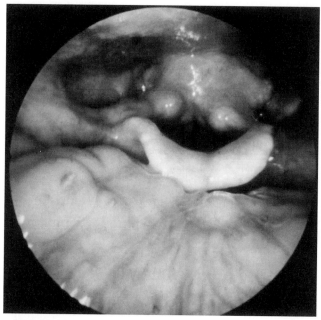

FIGURE 9–2
Acute laryngitis: interarytenoid edema prevents complete glottal closure.

shouting, talking on the telephone, or speaking over loud noises. Talking with laryngitis is like continuing to hike when the shoes have worn blisters on the feet. Coughing and throat clearing can also contribute to the injury. All patients should be instructed to avoid throat clearing. Guaifenesin, a mucolytic expectorant, reduces the urge to clear the throat and improves lubrication of the vocal folds. If the patient has an irritative, nonproductive cough, then cough suppressant medication is indicated. Steroids are not recommended in the routine management of laryngitis. Although they generally provide prompt temporary improvement in symptoms, they can actually contribute to injury of the larynx: The edema is resolved and so the patient feels better and talks more; however, the injury has not healed and the patient has lost important feedback cues that would normally limit overuse of the voice. Steroids are indicated only when the patient has an urgent, short-term need to use the voice and when examination rules out ulceration or bleeding of the larynx. Patients must be carefully instructed to limit voice use and should be closely monitored.

If the patient has an URI, a sympathomimetic decongestant such as pseudoephedrine is useful not only in relieving nasal obstruction but also in reducing laryngeal edema. Over-the-counter antihistamines should be avoided because they lead to thicker mucus and drying of the vocal folds. Antibiotics should be used only if a bacterial infection, such as sinusitis, is suspected.

If gastroesophageal reflux is implicated, then acid suppression is indicated. First-line management would include the use of an H_2 blocker, such as cimetidine or ranitidine. If the patient is already taking such medication, or if first-line therapy fails, a proton pump inhibitor should be prescribed. Gastric motility–enhancing medication may also be required.

When to Refer

Acute onset of hoarseness is most often due to benign laryngitis. However, in some cases, hoarseness requires immediate attention by an otolaryngologist. Sudden hoarseness that occurs during extreme vocal effort or heavy lifting may be due to bleeding into the vocal fold. Hoarseness due to external trauma may represent a laryngeal fracture. Hoarseness after endotracheal intubation is usually due to mild edema and inflammation, but if hoarseness is severe or if there is significant pain, immediate consultation is indicated.

When hoarseness lasts more than 2 weeks and does not respond to appropriate medical management, the larynx should be examined by an otolaryngologist. This is particularly true for two groups of patients. In smokers, laryngeal cancer is a significant concern. In young children, chronic hoarseness may be due to laryngeal papilloma, which could progress to airway obstruction.

KEY POINTS

— Diagnosis is primarily by history, as physical signs are often subtle.

— Treatment is primarily supportive, allowing spontaneous resolution.

— Voice rest permits healing.

— If gastroesophageal reflux is implicated, acid suppression is indicated.

— Steroids are rarely indicated for acute laryngitis and can result in exacerbation.

Suggested Reading

Woodson GE. Hoarseness and laryngitis. In Rakel R (ed.): *Conn's Current Therapy.* Philadelphia: WB Saunders, 1998, pp 29–31.

Chronic Laryngitis

Chronic laryngitis may result from persistence of acute laryngitis or may develop gradually over time. The most common contributing factors are essentially the same as for acute laryngitis: acid reflux, vocal abuse, and URI. In patients with chronic laryngitis, an acute URI may have been a precipitating event. Chronic sinusitis may be implicated in perpetuating chronic laryngeal inflammation.

Presentation

A patient with chronic laryngitis always sounds hoarse, and many have frequent episodes of superimposed acute infection, with sudden exacerbation of symptoms. The voice is rough, and the patient notes that speaking involves increased effort. As with acute laryngitis, pain may or may not be present, and airway symptoms are usually absent.

Diagnosis

Diagnosis is based on a history of a long-term vocal impairment and the physical findings of laryngeal inflammation. In addition, almost all patients have developed abnormal laryngeal posture during speech, either as a cause or result of the inflammation. Some patients speak by approximating the false vocal folds. Other patients "squeeze" the larynx during speech, shortening the vocal folds and compressing the larynx in the anteroposterior dimension. An important component of diagnosis is to rule out other causes of chronic hoarseness. Laryngeal cancer is a significant concern, particularly in patients who smoke and drink heavily. It is also important to detect benign lesions, such as polyps or nodules, which are treatable causes of hoarseness. This may require the use of stroboscopy, particularly if the lesion is subglottic or submucosal. If the larynx appears to be normal on physical examination, then a psychogenic or neurogenic voice disorder should be suspected.

Natural History

Chronic laryngitis is usually a stationary disability that exists for many years without progression. However, if gastroesophageal reflux is a contributing factor, then inflammation can be more severe. Mucosal ulceration can lead to long-term complications, such as joint fixation, vocal fold scarring, or subglottic stenosis. In addition, the risk of laryngeal cancer is significantly higher in patients with chronic reflux laryngitis. In the vast majority of patients with laryngeal cancer, the tumor can be attributed to smoking. But among those who do not smoke, acid reflux laryngitis appears to play a major role.

Treatment

All patients with chronic laryngitis need voice therapy to eliminate maladaptive behaviors and vocal abuse. Contributing factors such as reflux and infection should be controlled medically.

When to Refer

An otolaryngologist should examine all patients who have chronic hoarseness.

KEY POINTS

— Etiologic factors are the same as for acute laryngitis: vocal abuse, infection, and reflux.

— Reflux laryngitis should be treated aggressively because it increases the risk of laryngeal cancer and can result in laryngeal scarring.

— Physical examination of the larynx is essential to rule out cancer or benign lesion.

Vocal Nodules

Vocal nodules are calluses on the vocal folds. They result from vocal abuse: talking too loudly, too much, and with improper vocal technique. Nodules occur frequently in young children and cheerleaders, and are an occupational hazard for singers and grade-school teachers. In some singers, small nodules have no impact on the voice and may actually serve a protective role. Figure 9–3 is a diagram of a vocal nodule.

Presentation

Patients with vocal nodules have a raspy voice and often report frequent bouts of laryngitis. Children may be noted to have a deep, "froggy" voice. Singers may note that they have a reduced vocal range, with difficulty in reaching high notes, and require a longer warm-up period before singing.

Diagnosis

Clinical history is not sufficient to establish the diagnosis, but it is important to identify the factors contributing to nodule formation. Vocally demanding situations should be identified, such as cheerleading or speaking over loud noises. Occasionally, nodules develop because of severe coughing.

Diagnosis is established by physical examination of the larynx, using mirror examination or office endoscopy. The appearance is so

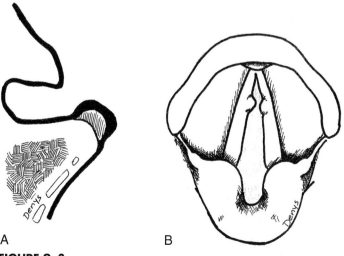

A   B

FIGURE 9–3
Diagram of vocal nodule, **A,** coronal section, **B,** view from above.

characteristic that an experienced examiner can confidently rule out malignancy as a consideration. Nodules appear as symmetric swelling on both vocal folds, at the midpoint of the membranous portion. In other words, they are characteristically located halfway between the anterior commissure and the vocal process of the arytenoid cartilage (Fig. 9–4). Nodules are almost always symmetric, so that significant asymmetry strongly suggests another pathology. The size and consistency of nodules vary considerably, from subtle swelling, noted only on stroboscopy, to large exophytic masses. In early stages, nodules are edemetous and soft, but with maturity they become cornified and firm, with thickened epithelium. They may occasionally be large and polypoid.

It is helpful to videotape or photograph the lesions, so that progress and response to treatment can be objectively monitored. Voice recording and analysis is helpful to document the severity of hoarseness and to follow response to treatment. However, the diagnosis is primarily based on findings on physical examination, not analysis of the voice.

In children, physical examination in the office may be difficult. If so, direct laryngoscopy under general anesthesia is required to establish the diagnosis and rule out the possibility of laryngeal papilloma.

Natural History

Nodules produce a gradually progressive decrease in vocal quality and endurance. Frequent episodes of acute laryngitis are common. In children, nodules commonly regress spontaneously during puberty,

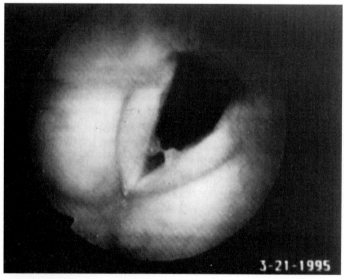

FIGURE 9–4
Vocal nodules.

particularly in boys. In adults, nodules eventually stabilize as a chronic and persisting vocal disability, unless the patient undergoes successful treatment or has a significant lifestyle change.

Treatment

The cornerstone of treatment is voice therapy. Voice restriction or rest can often result in temporary improvement. However, the crucial clinical objective is to identify and eliminate abusive vocal behavior. If vocal habits are corrected, nodules nearly always resolve. This process may require weeks or months. Occasionally, early surgical removal may be recommended, to hasten recovery of a normal voice. However, if the underlying vocal problem is not corrected, the nodules are very likely to recur. Moreover, surgery carries the risk of permanent vocal impairment due to scarring. Therefore voice therapy is the initial treatment of choice. The major difficulty in managing care of these patients is that insurance carriers are frequently unaware of the need for voice therapy and will not reimburse such treatment. It is in the best interests of both the patient and the third-party payer to vigorously appeal any denial of payment. Voice therapy is much more cost effective than surgery and avoids the risks of surgical complications.

Surgery should be reserved for persisting lesions that are symptomatic. Treatment is thus based on vocal function, not on the appearance of the vocal folds. There are generally two scenarios in which surgery is needed: Sometimes the vocal nodules are so large or firm that they are not reversible. In other cases, the lesion is actually not a nodule at all but a submucosal cyst, which can be treated only by surgical excision.

When to Refer

All patients with chronic hoarseness should be examined by an otolaryngologist.

KEY POINTS

— Vocal nodules are diagnosed by physical examination.

— Voice therapy is the treatment of choice.

— Surgery is indicated only when nodules do not resolve with voice therapy and the patient is still hoarse.

Suggested Reading

Murry T, Woodson GE. A comparison of three methods for the management of vocal fold nodules. *J Voice* 6:271–276, 1992.

Vocal Fold Polyps

Vocal fold polyps are soft-tissue masses on the membranous vocal fold. They may be sessile or pedunculated. They appear to be out-pouching of mucosa, distended by edema and loose stroma (Fig. 9–5). The cause is unknown; however, in some patients, polyps have been observed to develop after bleeding into the vocal fold, implicating degeneration of a hematoma as a potential cause.

Some authors assert that it is difficult to distinguish between a vocal fold polyp and a nodule and argue that all should be referred to as "bumps." It is true that there are no distinguishing histologic features of these lesions, and virtually any benign laryngeal tissue sent to the pathologist is likely to be diagnosed as a nodule. However, the vast majority of laryngologists concur that nodules can be distinguished from polyps on the basis of findings on physical examination. The importance of making this distinction is that optimal clinical management is quite different in the two disorders.

Presentation

Occasionally, a polyp may be noted incidentally during a routine laryngeal examination. Most often, however, the patient presents with chronic hoarseness. If the polyp is large, there may be associated dyspnea.

Diagnosis

Lesions are detected on physical examination of the larynx. Excisional biopsy is required if a tumor or other pathologic process is suspected.

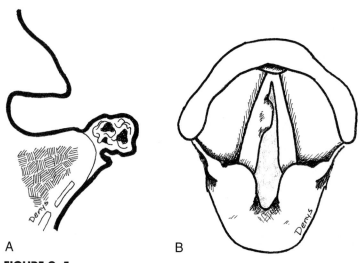

A   B

FIGURE 9–5
Diagram of vocal polyp, **A,** coronal section, **B,** view from above.

The histologic appearance of a polyp is rather nonspecific. Therefore, the distinction between a nodule and a polyp is made clinically, on the basis of findings on physical examination of the larynx. Polyps are generally smooth and pale (Fig. 9–6). If the polyp is very erythematous or has an uneven or rough surface, another pathology should be suspected, such as laryngeal papilloma or cancer.

Natural History

Most patients with laryngeal polyps have chronic hoarseness. Recurring bouts of acute laryngitis are common, because prolonged talking involves repetitive collisions between the polyp and both vocal folds. Polyps usually remain stable in size, but bleeding can cause a sudden increase in size, even to the point of occluding the airway. The risk of developing cancer in a polyp is very low. Polyps do not regress, but it is not unusual for a patient to cough out a pendunculated polyp.

Treatment

If the lesion's appearance suggests papilloma or cancer, then the lesion should be excised for histologic evaluation. If the patient has little or no hoarseness and the lesion clearly appears to be benign, then clinical observation is reasonable, with repeated laryngeal exam-

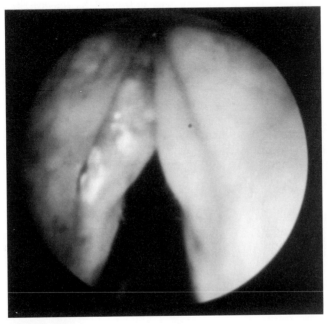

FIGURE 9–6
Vocal fold polyp.

inations. Most of the time, patients do have hoarseness; sometimes there is even airway distress. In such cases, polyps should be removed transorally under general anesthesia, using suspension microlaryngoscopy. The minimum possible amount of tissue should be excised. Voice therapy is often quite helpful in rehabilitation.

When to Refer

Any patient with chronic hoarseness or laryngeal lesions should be referred to an otolaryngologist.

KEY POINTS

— Laryngeal polyps cause hoarseness and sometimes airway obstruction.

— Polyps should be surgically excised if they cause symptoms or if the physical appearance suggests a tumor.

— Some pedunculated polyps auto-amputate and are expectorated.

Contact Ulcer and Granuloma

Laryngeal ulcers and granulomas typically appear on the vocal process of the arytenoid cartilage, the posterior portion of the vocal fold (Fig. 9–7). Because this is a point of constant contact and maximal pressure during phonation, these lesions are referred to as contact

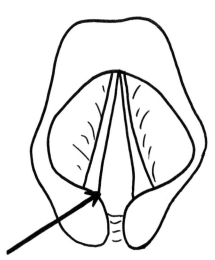

FIGURE 9–7
Location of a contact granuloma or ulcer.

ulcers and contact granulomas. Several factors have been implicated in the pathogenesis of contact granuloma, including vocal abuse, throat clearing, tracheal intubation, and gastroesophageal reflux.

Presentation

The most common presenting symptoms is hoarseness. Sore throat or a sensation of "something in the throat" is also frequently noted. The clinician will notice that many of these patients exhibit frequent throat clearing, an observation that can be confirmed by friends and family of the patient, yet few patients are aware of this as a symptom. Many of the patients will have vocally demanding occupations, such as preaching or litigating. In some, orotracheal intubation can be identified as the precipitating event for symptoms. Intubation-related granuloma is more often seen in women, probably because of the smaller size of the larynx. However, non–intubation related ulcer and granuloma is predominantly a disease of men.

Diagnosis

The medical history of a patient with a contact ulcer or granuloma is indistinguishable from that of a patient with chronic reflux laryngitis. Patients should be questioned about symptoms of reflux, including heartburn, belching, sour taste in the mouth, and water brash. To identify vocal abuse, patients should be asked about shouting, loud talking, frequent pain or loss of voice with prolonged speaking, and the need to speak often in a noisy environment.

These lesions are detected only by physical examination of the larynx. A granuloma is usually easily seen as an exophytic mass on the vocal process (Fig. 9–8). However, an ulcer is more difficult to detect, particularly when it is tiny. Diagnosis is best established by rigid office videoendoscopy, which permits careful evaluation of an enlarged image of the larynx. Flexible endoscopy is also useful, to identify abusive laryngeal posture during connected speech.

Natural History

Reflux is probably a lifelong problem for these patients, existing prior to the development of the lesion and continuing after its resolution. Untreated gastroesophageal reflux has been identified as a risk factor for the development of laryngeal cancer. Therefore, these patients should be followed carefully over the long term. Most will require long-term acid suppression.

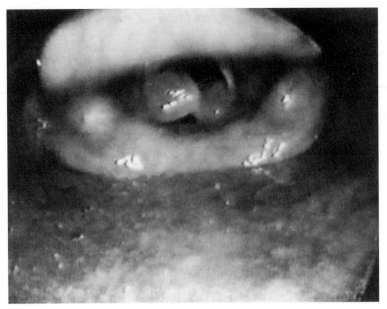

FIGURE 9–8
Contact granuloma.

Treatment

Treatment is medical control of the factors contributing to laryngeal inflammation. Gastoresophageal reflux has long been regarded as a causative factor for these lesions, but until recent years, there has been little evidence to support the efficacy of reflux management. The advent of proton pump inhibitor medication, which profoundly suppresses acid secretion, has finally provided an effective treatment. Omeprazole (20 mg/day) or levamisole (30 mg/day) is extremely effective relieving symptoms in most patients within 4–6 weeks, although complete resolution of the lesion may require several months. If clinical improvement is not noted within the first 4–6 weeks, the dose of proton pump inhibitor may be doubled and/or a gastric motility enhancer may be prescribed. It is important to note that acid suppression is effective even in patients with no clinical history of reflux symptoms.

Patients should be instructed in basic reflux precautions. They should not eat or drink for 2 hours before bedtime and should avoid foods that stimulate acid production.

Patients should also be counseled in vocal hygiene. They should avoid throat clearing and vocally demanding behavior, such as speaking during loud ambient noise or shouting. If vocal abuse is clearly identified, then patients should received concomitant voice therapy.

Medication should be continued for at least 2 months after resolution of the lesions, and then a trial of less stringent acid management may be attempted, stepping the patient down to H_2-blocker medication. Most patients require some form of chronic treatment because reflux is a lifelong problem. In patients with severe and persisting disease, gastric fundoplication should be considered.

For those patients whose lesions do not completely resolve and who continue to have symptoms, botulinum toxin treatment should be considered, to decrease the force of vocal fold closure. The rationale is that by preventing the trauma induced by coughing, throat clearing, and loud phonation, healing can occur. The toxin is injected directly into the vocal fold, percutaneously or transorally. This approach is not widely used, but it seems to be effective. The disadvantage is that it does reduce vocal power for a few months.

Direct laryngoscopy with biopsy is indicated if the appearance of the lesion suggests a tumor. Surgery should also be considered for a persistent granuloma that is symptomatic. There is an extremely high rate of recurrence after surgical excision. Surgery also carries risks of anesthetic complications and scarring. Therefore, it should be reserved for lesions that do not respond to medical management. If the diagnosis has been established and the lesion is asymptomatic, surgery is not indicated. Medical management should be continued, with semiannual laryngeal examination.

When to Refer

All patients with contact ulcers or granulomas should be referred to an otolaryngologist.

KEY POINTS

— Gastroesophageal reflux plays a role in all patients with contact lesions of the larynx, even when there is no history of reflux symptoms.

— Contact granuloma is fairly easy to detect on physical examination, whereas diagnosis of ulcer often requires office endoscopy.

— Primary treatment is medical management of reflux.

— Reduction of vocal fold trauma is also important, by voice therapy or injection of botulinum toxin into laryngeal muscles.

— Most patients require long-term acid suppression.

— Direct laryngoscopy is indicated when histologic diagnosis is needed or when the lesion fails to respond to medical therapy and the patient still has symptoms.

Suggested Reading

Wani M, Woodson GE. Laryngeal contact granuloma. *Laryngoscope* 109:1589–1593, 1999.

Papilloma

Laryngeal papilloma is an exophytic mucosal mass (Fig. 9–9). There are usually multiple lesions. Most often, they arise from the squamous mucosa on the membranous vocal fold but can involve any portion of the respiratory tract. In fact, a widely accepted term for this disorder is *recurrent respiratory papillomatosis*. This term also indicates an important clinical feature: the high rate of recurrence after surgical removal.

A virus, the same virus that causes venereal warts, causes laryngeal papilloma. Children with respiratory papillomatosis have acquired the disease from mothers with venereal warts. At one time, it was believed that the virus was acquired during passage through the birth canal; however, children can acquire the disease even when delivered by cesarean section. Thus, it is now believed that the virus is transmitted hematogenously in utero. Immunologic studies indicate a high rate of transmission of the virus to babies of mothers with genital warts, yet only about 1% of infected babies actually develop respiratory papillomatosis. The factors that determine which children will develop the disease remain to be elucidated.

It has been demonstrated that the virus infects cells throughout the respiratory tract and that the majority of infected cells appear to be grossly normal. Thus, when the visible lesion is removed, a new papilloma can grow in its place from cells in which infection had been latent.

Presentation

Laryngeal papilloma is manifested differently in adults and children. Adults most often have isolated lesions with a lower rate of recurrence,

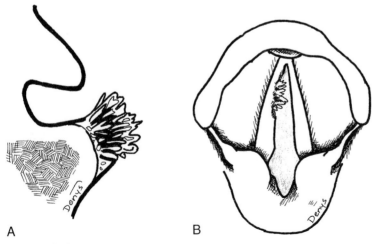

A   B

FIGURE 9–9
Diagram of a papilloma, **A,** coronal section, **B,** view from above.

and symptoms are restricted to hoarseness. In children, the severity of the disease varies, but in general, lesions are more diffuse and recurrence occurs more rapidly than in adults. Although hoarseness is the initial presentation in children, the most serious problem is airway obstruction, as the laryngeal lesions become so large that they occlude the lumen (Fig. 9–10). In the most severe cases, the lower respiratory tract is also involved by papillomatosis.

Diagnosis

Diagnosis can only be conclusively established by histologic examination of an excised lesion. However, the gross appearance of the lesion is usually fairly characteristic (Fig. 9–11). Thus, the key to diagnosis is physical examination of the larynx in patients with a history of hoarseness.

Because of the potentially serious nature of the disease in children, any young child with hoarseness should be presumed to have papillomatosis until proven otherwise. Laryngeal mirror examination can be quite problematic in children, but the use of flexible endoscopy permits adequate office examination of all but the most difficult patients. If the larynx cannot be adequately inspected in the office, then direct laryngoscopy under general anesthesia is indicated. If a child not only is hoarse but also has stridor or difficulty breathing, however mild, then there is a significant danger of impending airway obstruction and surgical endocscopy is indicated as soon as possible.

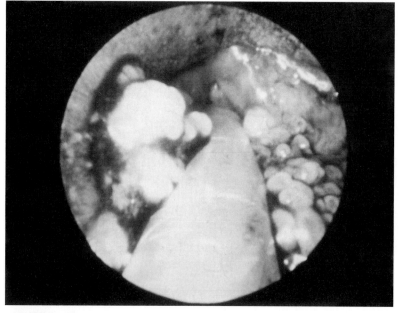

FIGURE 9–10
Obstructing laryngeal papilloma. Note endotracheal tube and laryngoscope blade.

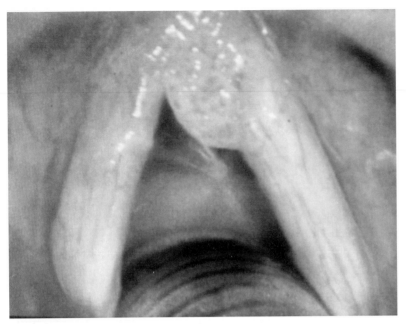

FIGURE 9–11
Focal laryngeal papilloma in an adult.

Natural History

Hoarseness is the initial presenting symptom, caused by interference of vocal fold vibration by the mass lesion on the vocal fold. As the lesion becomes larger, hoarseness becomes more severe. Airway obstruction by papilloma is very rare in adults but is a significant problem in children. Figure 9–10 demonstrates the appearance at laryngoscopy of a child whose airway distress gradually progressed to near total airway obstruction. The disease is usually much more indolent in adults, in whom lesions may remain stable for long periods of time. Development of malignancy is a rare occurrence.

Treatment

The mainstay of treatment is surgical ablation or excision of symptomatic lesions. Laser vaporization has become a popular tool for treating papilloma; however, it is important to submit a representative sample of tissue for histologic examination. If the lesion is small or well circumscribed, complete surgical excision is often preferable, as this permits optimal healing and recovery of vocal function. With repeated recurrences, surgical scarring becomes an increasing concern, as scarring can impair the voice as well as the airway. Thus, repeat surgical excisions should be planned not on the physical appearance of recurrent lesions but on functional impairment. In other words, surgery should be undertaken to maintain the voice and the airway, not to remove every identifiable lesion. In adults, the voice is the chief consideration, whereas in children, surgery should be performed with sufficient frequency to maintain the airway. Tracheotomy should be avoided if at all possible.

In some patients, the disease is so diffuse or recurs so rapidly that surgical control is unsatisfactory. In these cases, adjuvant therapy is indicated. Interferon has been shown to be frequently effective in decreasing the recurrence rate. Because of its toxicity, it is recommended only for patients with severe disease. Indole-3-carbinol, a dietary supplement found in cruciferous vegetables, has been shown to have some ameliorative effect on the disease. It has virtually no toxicity and is usually quite well tolerated; for this reason, it could be considered for any patient with papilloma. However, it is much less effective than is interferon. Intralesional injection of a new antiviral drug, cidofovir, has been demonstrated by clinical trials in Belgium to be quite effective. This treatment is currently under investigation in the United States and holds considerable promise.

When to Refer

Any patient with a lesion of the vocal fold should be referred to an otolaryngologist.

KEY POINTS

— Any child with hoarseness should be presumed to have laryngeal papilloma until proven otherwise.

— Laryngeal papillomatosis can cause airway obstruction in children.

— Diagnosis requires histologic examination of excised tissue.

— Recurrences are extremely common, and repeat surgery should be planned to maximize function.

— Recurrent asymptomatic lesions need not be excised.

— Interferon treatment is indicated for severe recurrent disease with airway compromise.

— Avoid tracheotomy if at all possible.

Suggested Reading

Rosen CA, Woodson GE, Thompson JWT, Hengesteg AP. Preliminary results of the use of indole-3 for recurrent respiratory papillomatosis. *Otolaryngol Head Neck Surg* 18:810–815, 1998.

Cysts and Sulci

Sometimes very small malformations of the vocal fold can cause significant hoarseness. Included in this category are submocosal cysts and invaginations of epithelium, referred to as sulci. Another form of sulcus is the partial absence of the submuocosal connective tissue that normally separates the epithelium from the underlying vocal ligament. Figure 9–12 shows the structure of these lesions.

There appears to be considerable variation in the incidence of these lesions, probably according to ethnic or racial differences. For example, sulci are commonly encountered in South America and parts of Europe but are much less frequent in the general U.S. population.

The precise cause is not known. They may be congenital lesions or the result of injury to the vocal fold, sustained by vocal abuse. A small sulcus may result from rupture of a cyst, with marsupialization.

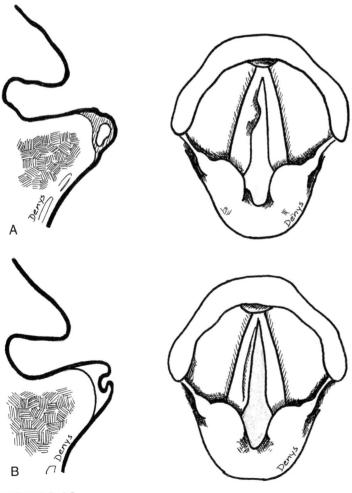

FIGURE 9-12
Vocal fold: **A,** cyst and **B,** sulci.

Presentation

Although these lesions are very small and difficult to detect clinically, they can profoundly impair vocal function. Patients present with a weak voice, easy vocal fatigue, and sometimes frequent bouts of laryngitis.

Diagnosis

Large cysts may be visible on routine laryngeal examination; however, most cysts and sulci cannot be detected on routine examination. Stroboscopy is often helpful in revealing small cysts (Fig. 9–13), but direct laryngoscopy is usually required to detect sulci and many cysts.

Natural History

Little is known about the natural history of these lesions. Many affected patients have a history of lifelong hoarseness, suggesting that the lesions are congenital. This is particularly true for large sulci; however, some cysts appear to be acquired, perhaps due to the entrapment of epithelium after trauma. The presumed mechanism of trauma is vocal abuse. Small sulci may develop from ruptured cysts. Most sulci appear to be stable, nonprogressive lesions, whereas cysts have been observed to enlarge.

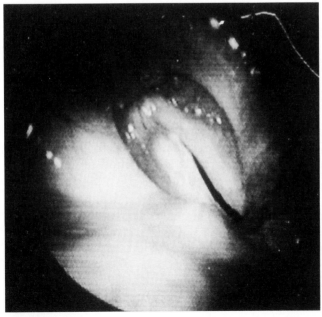

FIGURE 9–13
Vocal fold cyst.

Treatment

Voice therapy can optimize vocal function but will not result in regression of the lesion. Surgical treatment offers the only possibility of cure and it is usually quite beneficial to remove cysts. However, postoperative scarring may result in poor function. Surgical treatment of sulci is less effective because most lesions involve a deficiency of submucosal tissue that cannot be replaced. In most cases, vocal function will remain poor, with no effective treatment.

When to Refer

All patients with chronic hoarseness should be evaluated by a laryngologist, even when no pathology can be identified on office laryngoscopy.

KEY POINTS

— Even when the larynx appears totally normal on physical examination, there may be significant functional impairment by submucosal pathology.

— Submucosal cysts can be treated with surgical excision, whereas surgery for sulci is less often effective.

Suggested Reading

Zwirner P, Murry T, Woodson GE. Phonatory function of neurologically impaired patients. *J Commun Disord* 24:287–300, 1991.

Laryngeal Aging

An inevitable part of aging is some degree of decrement in vocal function. This is due to a number of processes that occur in the larynx with old age. The thyroid cartilage becomes ossified and therefore less resonant and "tuned" to higher frequencies. The vocal ligament loses elasticity, so that the vocal fold tends to bow and sag. The vocalis muscle atrophies, so that the vocal fold is thinner (Fig. 9–14). In postmenopausal women, the submucosal connective tissue on the vibratory edge of the vocal fold becomes edemetous. When this edema becomes extreme, most commonly in smokers, the entire vocal fold appears polypoid (Fig. 9–14).

A second factor in vocal aging is the decrease in pulmonary reserve. As the available expiratory volume decreases, the capacity to shout and speak loudly diminishes.

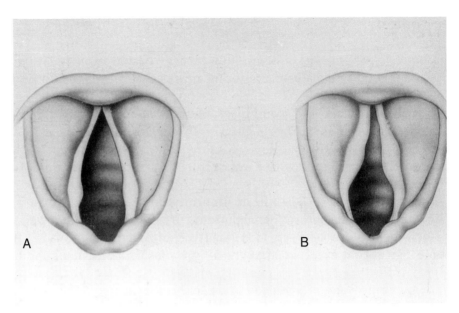

FIGURE 9–14
Age-related changes in the larynx: **A,** male; **B,** female. (Reproduced with permission from Close L, Woodson CF. Common upper airway disorders in the elderly. *Geriatrics* 44:67–72, 1989. Copyright by Advanstar Communications Inc. Advanstar Communications Inc. retains all rights to this article.)

Presentation

Typically, the voice of an older person is weaker and thinner. Patients have difficulty communicating because they cannot make themselves understood. In men, the voice pitch becomes higher, owing to ossification of the thyroid cartilage and atrophy of the vocalis muscle. In women, however, the effects of vocal fold thinning are offset to varying degrees by edema, and in many women the voice becomes deep and husky. With extreme edema, the airway may be compromised. This is a particular problem in women who have been heavy smokers, as pulmonary function may also be impaired.

Diagnosis

The sound of an aging voice is easy to recognize. Laryngeal examination should be performed to rule out other lesions and to confirm that the voice changes are due to aging and not to some other pathology.

Natural History

Vocal aging is highly variable. In general, the effects of aging are less in people who are robust and active, and the best-preserved voices are seen in singers who continue to sing regularly.

Treatment

The majority of patients are satisfied by the reassurance that their vocal changes are a part of the aging process. However, some find their vocal impairment to be quite frustrating and feel that it interferes with their work and social interaction. For such motivated individuals, it is reasonable to try to improve the voice as much as possible.

The first step is voice therapy, to increase loudness and breath support. This probably works by restoring strength and bulk to atrophic muscles. It has been shown that resistance training can significantly increase the bulk of limb muscles in elderly subjects. With such physical therapy, some patients previously reliant on walkers or wheelchairs achieve significantly improved ambulation. It seems logical that exercise of laryngeal muscles could have a similar salutary effect.

If the improvement achieved by voice therapy is insufficient, then surgical augmentation of the vocal folds is an option. Vocal fold bulk can be restored by injection of fat or collagen. This is accomplished by either direct laryngoscopy under general anesthesia or by percutaneous or transoral injection in the office using endoscopic guidance. If more substantial improvement in glottic closure is needed, a medialization thyroplasty may be performed, via an external incision in the neck.

When to Refer

Age-related voice changes are nearly universal. Therefore, not every patient with a weak or quavering voice needs a laryngeal examination. However, when the patient desires improvement or when the handicap interferes with work or social interaction, then laryngologic consultation is appropriate. Patients should also be referred for a laryngeal examination when the voice changes are atypical, suggesting pathology.

When laryngeal aging in women leads to airway compromise, consultation is urgently indicated.

KEY POINTS

— Vocal changes are a natural part of aging.

— Treatment is available for those who are motivated to improve the voice.

— Voice therapy is the initial treatment of choice.

— Surgery can be performed if voice therapy fails to achieve sufficient improvement.

Suggested Reading

Close L, Woodson GE. Common upper airway disorders in the elderly. *Geriatrics* 44:67–72, 1989.

Laryngeal Neuropathy

Damage to the nerves supplying the larynx can cause paralysis (Fig. 9–15) or weakness of the vocal folds, and in rare cases, episodic laryngospasm. When the vagus nerve is the site of the lesion, there is frequently associated paralysis of the pharynx and occasionally the soft palate as well. Injury to the recurrent laryngeal nerve rarely results in complete paralysis, even when the nerve is totally transected. This is because the nerve has a very strong capacity for regeneration. Unfortunately, nerve regeneration rarely results in usable function, because the nerve fibers often become jumbled and supply the wrong muscles. This results in synkinesis, analagous to the mass movement of the face that often occurs after Bell's palsy.

Laryngeal nerves may be damaged by surgical trauma, most commonly during thyroidectomy or cervical spine surgery. Less commonly, carotid endarterectomy is associated with laryngeal paralysis. Intubation alone can result in temporary paralysis. Thyroid tumors can compress or invade either recurrent laryngeal nerve. Lung cancer metastatic to mediastinal nodes can invade the left recurrent laryngeal nerve. Sometimes no reason can be found for the paralysis. It is widely assumed that many idiopathic neuropathies are due to viral infection.

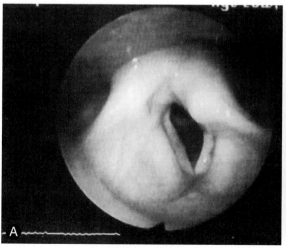 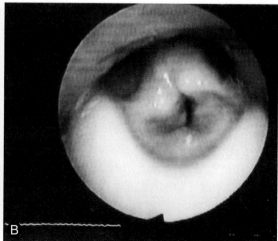

FIGURE 9–15
Vocal fold paralysis: **A,** inspiration; **B,** phonation.

Presentation

The symptoms of laryngeal nerve injury vary. Some patients with a completely immobile vocal fold have no symptoms whatsoever. Most often, unilateral laryngeal neuropathy results in hoarseness. If the nerve injury is complete, there is often associated dysphagia and aspiration, particularly if the vagus nerve is involved. When both sides of the larynx are paralyzed, breathing is impaired.

Diagnosis

Laryngeal neuropathy is suspected in a patient with a breathy voice and confirmed by examination of the larynx. Most cases of laryngeal paralysis can be detected on mirror examination, but more subtle weakness is difficult to appreciate by this technique. Flexible laryngoscopy is the best means of accurately assessing mobility of the larynx.

When laryngeal neuropathy is detected, it is essential to determine the cause. Sometimes the cause is obvious from the history, such as recent surgery or trauma. If not, then the patient should be assumed to have a tumor until it is proven otherwise. Progressive nerve compression by a tumor usually results in the gradual onset of a breathy voice; however, symptoms may also appear suddenly. A minimal workup would be a chest x-ray and a careful physical examination of the head and neck. At least one study has suggested that this is sufficient and is a cost-effective approach. Nevertheless, the consequences of missing an occult tumor are grave. For example, a malignant thyroid tumor may not be paplpable on physical examination, owing to location substernally or posteriorly. Metastasis to a subclavian node can also occur, and breast cancer can metastasize directly to the laryngeal nerves. Therefore, most laryngologists would recommend imaging of the entire course of the recurrent laryngeal nerve, with computed tomography or magnetic resonance imaging from the arch of the aorta to the base of the skull.

Natural History

An acute lesion of the recurrent laryngeal nerve results in a flaccid paralysis, with a large glottal gap on phonation. The voice is quite breathy. Over time, there are varying degrees of reinnervation, but usable motion rarely occurs. Instead, the paralyzed vocal fold gradually moves toward the midline, owing to the pull of reinnervated muscles. With this change in position, the normal vocal fold can better approximate the paralyzed one, so that the voice improves. In some patients, no other treatment is needed, but more often, the voice is still not strong enough. Figure 9–15 shows a larynx with a unilateral paralysis. Note that the paralyzed fold appears shorter. With phonation, the normal vocal fold is able to close the glottis, but this requires increased effort.

In a gradually progressive lesion, symptoms come on more slowly. Most often, gradual onset is due to involvement by tumor, and in such cases, reinnervation is extremely unlikely.

Treatment

Treatment is based on the patient's symptoms and the likelihood of spontaneous recovery. If there is a chance of recovery, then it is best to avoid permanent surgical therapy for at least 6 months. Voice therapy is helpful in optimizing vocal function. In some patients, it is helpful to inject absorbable gelatin foam to medialized the paralyzed vocal fold while waiting for spontaneous recovery. This can temporarily restore considerable function.

For many years, injection of Teflon paste was accepted as the treatment of choice for unilateral laryngeal paralysis. However, this fails to correct the flaccid, lateral vocal fold. Additionally, it is now recognized that there is a high incidence of granulomatous response to injected Teflon. In many cases, this granuloma is large enough to compromise the airway. Therefore, Teflon has fallen out of favor and is used primarily in patients whose paralysis is due to malignancy and whose life expectancy is short.

Current options include injecting fat or collagen into the vocal fold, placing an implant through the neck to medialize the fold (thyroplasty), or repositioning the arytenoid to place the paralyzed vocal fold in optimal position. The appropriate technique is selected on the basis of the glottic defect and the severity of symptoms.

When to Refer

All patients suspected of having laryngeal paralysis should be examined by an otolaryngologist.

KEY POINTS

— Laryngeal nerve injury is primarily manifested by a weak and breathy voice.

— Laryngeal paralysis may be the presenting sign of an occult tumor; thus, it is essential to carefully search for the cause.

— Permanent surgical treatment should usually be deferred for at least 6 months.

— Definitive treatment is dependent on the patient's symptoms and the configuration of the glottic gap.

Suggested Reading

Woodson GE, Miller RH. The timing of surgical intervention in laryngeal paralysis. *Otolaryngol Head Neck Surg* 89:294–297, 1981.

Spasmodic Dysphonia

In patients with spasmodic dysphonia, the voice is disrupted by frequent involuntary spasms of laryngeal muscle. The disorder was first described clinically more than a century ago, but until the 1970s, it was widely regarded to be a psychiatric problem. It is now generally accepted that spasmodic dysphonia is a central neurologic movement disorder. Specifically, it is considered to be a focal dystonia of the larynx. Generalized dystonia, which impairs the function of many large muscles throughout the body, is a hereditary disorder with an identified gene locus. Localized dystonias include torticollis (wry-neck), blepharospasm (eye blinking), and writer's cramp (hand spasm). The defect appears to be in the brain stem, with inappropriate muscle response to feedback.

Presentation

The onset of this disorder is usually gradual. The patient notes occasional "catching" in the voice that gradually increases in frequency. Eventually, the catches become so frequent and sustained that the voice sounds strained and the patient finds it very difficult to speak. The problem is worse when the patient is under stress or speaking on the telephone. In many patients, the symptoms are isolated to spontaneous speech, and patients are able to perform other phonatory tasks with no problem, such as humming, singing, laughing, reciting, or speaking in falsetto. Every patient modifies his or her pattern of speech to compensate for the spasms, and there are many different modes of compensation. For example, some whisper, some speak in a high pitch, and some use neck muscles to tighten the larynx even more. These variations in symptoms promulgated, for so many years, the notion that spasmodic dysphonia patients were psychiatrically disturbed.

Many patients have associated neurologic symptoms, such as tremor, head bobbing, torticollis, or blepharospasm. Some patients have a family history of similar problems.

Diagnosis

The sound of a voice with spasmodic dysphonia has unique characteristics that are easily recognized by an experienced laryngologist or speech pathologist. The voice is strained, with variations in pitch and loudness and frequent "breaks" in the voice.

The diagnosis is confirmed by findings on physical examination. The larynx should be observed during connected speech, using flexible transnasal endoscopy. In spasmodic dysphonia, the larynx is anatomically normal, but there are involuntary spasms of laryngeal muscles during speech. In most patients, the spasms result in excess closure of the larynx, but in a small subset, the spasms pull the vocal folds apart, so that the voice suddenly becomes breathy. A fine laryngeal tremor (which may also involve the pharynx or soft palate) is frequently noted during speech. A careful neurologic examination is essential, to rule out other neurologic disorders, such as parkinsonism.

It is sometimes difficult to distinguish between a patient with spasmodic dysphonia and a patient with a psychogenic voice disorder. Many emotionally disturbed or even malingering patients can simulate the strained voice of spasmodic dysphonia. A careful interview is usually very helpful in detecting psychiatric problems. Also, distraction of the patient during the interview or endoscopic examination may unmask normal speech. However, the most important distinguishing feature is the presence of involuntary voice breaks in the patient with neurogenic spasmodic dysphonia. These breaks can be identified by the trained ear but are more reliably and objectively documented by acoustic analysis of a voice recording.

Natural History

Spasmodic dysphonia usually develops gradually over several months, but occasionally the onset is sudden, following an illness or stressful life event. It may remain stable over many years, or gradually progress in severity. Rarely, symptoms may abate for variable intervals, but complete spontaneous recovery has not been reported. In a few patients, spasmodic dysphonia is the first sign of a generalized dystonia, with development of spasms in other muscles. However, in the majority of patients with spasmodic dysphonia, the disease remains confined to the larynx.

Treatment

Currently, the most widely accepted treatment is the injection of minute quantities of botulinum toxin into laryngeal muscles. This may be accomplished by injecting through the anterior neck, using electromyogram guidance, or via the mouth, under endoscopic control. The dose must be individualized, and injections are repeated whenever symptoms begin to recur, usually in 4–6 months.

Voice therapy alone is considered to be ineffective by most clinicians, although success has been reported with an intensive vocal rehabilitation program. Voice therapy enhances the efficacy of botulinum toxin therapy, extending the duration between injections.

Other alternatives are available for patients who desire a more permanent solution. Surgical transection of the recurrent laryngeal nerve was the first treatment reported to be effective for this order. It is still a viable option for the severely affected patient. However, many patients have unsatisfactory results, such as a weak and breathy voice or recurrence of spasms. More recently, two innovative approaches have been studied but have not yet gained widespread acceptance: (1) recurrent laryngeal nerve resection in combination with transfer of another nerve (ansa cervicalis) to provide stable tonic activity to the laryngeal muscles and (2) limited resection of laryngeal muscle.

When to Refer

An otolaryngologist should evaluate all patients with severely symptomatic voice disorders. Neurologic consultation is also recommended whenever a neurogenic voice disorder is suspected.

KEY POINTS

— Spasmodic dysphonia is a neurogenic disorder characterized by strained speech.

— Although symptoms are exacerbated by stress, it is not a psychosomatic disorder.

— Currently, the most widely accepted treatment is injection of botulinum toxin.

— In some patients, the disorder progresses to a generalized dystonia.

Suggested Reading

Woodson GE. Spasmodic dysphonia. In Gates GE, (ed.): *Current Therapy in Otolaryngology, Head and Neck Surgery.* St. Louis: Mosby, 1998, pp 436–439.

Other Neurogenic Dysphonias

A number of other neurologic diseases can disrupt the voice, including parkinsonism, amyotrophic lateral sclerosis, multiple sclerosis, cerebellar disorders, Huntington's chorea, intention tremor, palatal myoclonus, and pseudobulbar palsy. The voice may be weak and tremulous or harsh and strained.

Diagnosis

Neurologic impairment should be suspected when the larynx appears anatomically normal but the voice and speech are significantly impaired. Altered vocal resonance, such as a hypernasal voice or a "hot potato" voice, are signs of disordered pharyngeal and palatal function and strongly suggest neurologic disease. Dysarthria, dysphagia, and drooling are also indicators of neurologic dysfunction.

When to Refer

Diagnosis requires a carefully elicited medical history and complete neurologic examination, preferably by a neurologist. In addition, documentation of laryngeal and upper airway dysfunction requires flexible transnasal endoscopy. Treatment varies according to the specific neurologic disorder.

KEY POINTS

— When the voice is significantly abnormal and the larynx appears to be structurally normal, a neurologic disorder should be considered.

— Dysarthria, resonance changes, and associated dysphagia are signs that suggest possible neruologic impairment.

— Adequate clinical evaluation of neurologic disorders of the upper airway require collaboration between a neurologist and an otolaryngologist.

Suggested Reading

Miller RH, Woodson GE. Neurological evaluation of the larynx and pharynx. In Johnson JT, Blitzer A, Ossoff RH, Thomas JR, (eds.): *AAO-HNS Instructional Courses.* St. Louis: CV Mosby; 3:39–44, 1990.

Psychogenic, Factitious, and Functional Dysphonia

The category of nonorganic voice disorders includes psychogenic problems, willful misuse of the voice by malingerers, and bad vocal habits. It is not surprising that psychiatric disorders could impair the voice, because the voice conveys emotion and is also profoundly affected by emotion and stress. It is also understandable that factitious hoarseness would be a very easy way to feign a disability. Habitual voice misuse is analogous to poor posture.

Diagnosis

When the voice is abnormal and there is no evidence of structural abnormality or neurologic dysfunction, the possibility of nonorganic disease must be considered. Differentiation among the three causes is frequently difficult, although some specific disorders are easy to identify.

Hysterical aphonia is believed to be a conversion reaction. Patients speak in a whisper but are able to cough strongly and perform a Valsalva's maneuver. *La belle indifference* is a characteristic of these patients, as they do not seem particularly curious about the cause of the problem or eager to be cured. Flexible endoscopy confirms that the vocal folds have no lesions and move normally with breathing and coughing. During speech, the larynx constricts to form the "whisper triangle," but the vocal folds are not opposed. Sometimes the patient can be distracted and bits of normal phonation may occur. Making the patient laugh, by telling a joke, can demonstrate normal laryngeal activity as well.

Some patients feign a strained voice, similar to that of spasmodic dysphonia. It is often extremely difficult to differentiate these patients from those with spasmodic dysphonia. However, patients with "pseudo spasmodic dysphonia" can usually be easily distracted by other tasks, so that some normal phonation slips out without their notice. The most helpful clinical feature, however, is the presence of voice "breaks" in patients with spasmodic dysphonia and the absence of such breaks in patients with pseudodysfunction.

When a patient has habitual dysphonia, it may be difficult to determine whether the problem is intentional. The best indicator is often the response to a trial of voice therapy. Patients with habitual dysphonia can usually correct their behavior during the therapy session but may have difficulty maintaining good habits between sessions. Those with psychogenic or factitious problems are more resistant to making changes during therapy.

Treatment

In patients with hysterical aphonia, minimal intervention is often quite effective. A statement that the larynx looks normal and that the voice will probably recover in 1 or 2 days often results in miraculous recovery. This is because the patient is given permission to recover without losing face. When this approach is ineffective, only psychiatric intervention is likely to restore the voice.

For other disorders, a trial of voice therapy is the best first step. If the patient makes progress, then voice therapy is likely to be effective, no matter what the cause. However, if patients do not make corrections in speech during trial therapy, psychiatric referral is indicated.

When to Refer

Every patient with chronic hoarseness or voice loss should be evaluated by an otolaryngologist. If a psychogenic disorder is suspected, the patient's condition should be evaluated by a psychiatrist.

10

DISORDERS OF UPPER AERODIGESTIVE FUNCTION

The human upper aerodigestive tract is anatomically and functionally complex because it must serve the conflicting functions of breathing and swallowing. The pharynx must remain patent during respiration yet collapse forcefully for propulsion during swallowing. The larynx must be open during breathing and must be closed and pulled anteriorly during swallowing.

Swallowing and breathing are far more complex in humans than in other animals because in nonhuman mammals, the pharynx is partitioned into alimentary and respiratory canals by interdigitation of the uvula and epiglottis. Food travels around the epiglottis and larynx to reach the esophagus; thus, some animals are able to continue breathing while feeding. In humans, the larynx descends after infancy so that the pharynx functions as a single large chamber (Fig. 10–1). Some authors

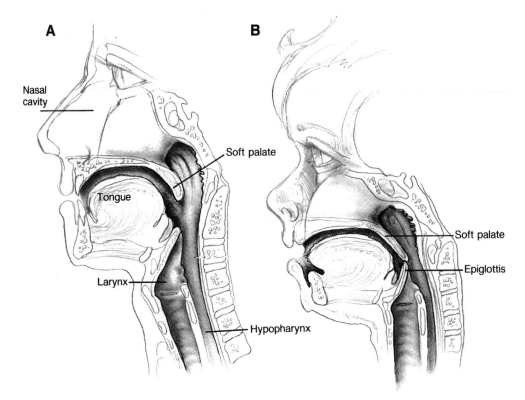

FIGURE 10-1
Maturational changes in the upper aerodigestive tract. **A,** Adult upper airway. Note lower position of larynx and gap between uvula and epiglottis. **B,** Diagram of the human infant upper airway, demonstrating interdigitation of the uvula and soft palate. (From Bailey BJ, Pagos A [eds]. *Head and Neck Surgery—Otolaryngology,* 2nd ed., Philadelphia: Lippincott Williams & Wilkins, 1998.)

have suggested that human infants are obligate nasal breathers and have the ability to swallow and breathe simultaneously. Recent research indicates that this is not the case. Infants do cease breathing during a swallow, and although they strongly prefer nasal breathing, normal babies are able to breathe orally.

A system this complex can be easily disrupted by motor weakness, sensory deficits, incoordination or spasm, or mechanical obstruction. Many diseases affect both breathing and swallowing, such as acutely swollen and infected tonsils or neuromuscular weakness.

Upper Airway Obstruction

Acute upper airway obstruction is a life-threatening medical emergency. This chapter deals with chronic upper airway obstruction, which is associated with an increased mortality rate and also has a significant impact on quality of life and overall health.

The upper airway may be impaired by mechanical obstruction or by failure of the mechanisms that normally maintain airway patency. The upper airway is subjected to negative pressure during inspiration. Without active dilation, collapse may occur at several levels. The genioglossus muscle pulls the tongue forward to prevent collapse of the base of the tongue into the pharynx. The hyoid bone is pulled upward and anteriorly to prevent collapse of the hypopharynx. The vocal folds abduct with each inspiration to reduce resistance. The palate must be positioned appropriately to permit either nasal or oral breathing.

Diagnosis

The diagnosis of upper airway obstruction is often missed because it is not included in the differential diagnosis of dyspnea. When a patient complains of difficulty in breathing, physicians frequently assume the problem to be pulmonary in origin. Failure to consider the possibility of upper airway obstruction can result in serious delay in treatment. For example, many patients with subglottic stenosis are treated for presumed asthma, until airway obstruction becomes sufficiently severe to constitute an emergency and the diagnosis becomes obvious. Whenever a patient presents with difficulty in breathing, the possibility of upper airway obstruction should be routinely considered.

Another source of difficulty in diagnosis stems from the fact that upper airway obstruction may be intermittent, as in episodic laryngospasm, or may occur during sleep. In either case, the physician is unable to observe the obstructive episodes and must rely on history gleaned from the patient and his or her family and friends.

Stridor is a key physical sign in upper airway obstruction. This may be either loud enough to be clearly audible to anyone in the same room or so mild that it is detected only by auscultation of the neck. Inspiratory stridor is characteristic of extrathoracic upper airway obstruction, at the level of the larynx, pharynx, or subglottic trachea. Inspiratory effort against a narrowed upper airway results in increasingly negative intraluminal pressure, tending to collapse the airway. Expiration is easier because the airway is pushed open by positive pressure. Obstruction of the intrathoracic trachea presents differently because the outer walls are subject to intrathoracic, rather than atmospheric pressure; thus, the stridor is biphasic. When the patient is fatigued, or when obstruction is especially severe, there may be no

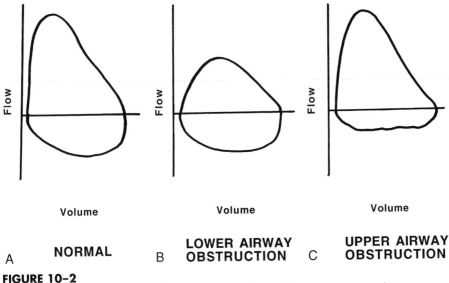

FIGURE 10-2
Flow–volume loop: **A,** normal; **B,** lower airway occlusion; **C,** upper airway occlusion.

audible stridor. Suprasternal and intercostal retractions during inspiration and the use of accessory inspiratory muscles are important indicators of the severity of obstruction.

The most useful screening test for fixed upper airway obstruction is spirometry. Standard test batteries are intended to evaluate pulmonary function, focusing on static lung volumes and expiratory flows. Extrathoracic obstruction of the upper airway preferentially affects inspiratory airflow. Thus, measures of peak inspiratory flow, as well as the flow–volume loop, will be abnormal in patients with laryngeal or upper tracheal stenosis and the inspiratory limb of the flow–volume loop will be characteristically flattened (Fig. 10–2). The situation is more complex when the patient also has pulmonary disease with significant depression of expiratory flow. Criteria have been established to aid in detecting extrathoracic upper airway dysfunction in these patients, as listed in Table 10–1. Obstruction of the intrathoracic trachea will affect both inspiratory and expiratory flow. Spirometry is not particularly helpful in patients with episodic upper airway obstruction.

TABLE 10-1 · **CRITERIA FOR THE DIAGNOSIS OF UPPER AIRWAY OBSTRUCTION**

$FIF_{50} \leq 100$ L/m
$FEF_{50}/FIF_{50} \geq 1$
$FEV_1/PEF \geq 10$ mL/min

FIF_{50} = forced inspiratory flow at 50% of vital capacity; FEF_{50} = forced expiratory flow at 50% of vital capacity; FEV_1 = forced expiratory volume at 1 minute; PEF = peak expiratory flow.

Advances in office endoscopy, imaging, and laboratory testing allow precise diagnosis of the location and nature of upper airway obstruction. Improved surgical techniques and better understanding of physiology offer better outcomes, yet there are still many problems that cannot be overcome, so that chronic tracheotomy is still necessary in many patients.

Obstructive Sleep Apnea

The most common organic cause of daytime somnolence is obstructive sleep apnea (OSA), affecting approximately 4% of men and 2% of women. Patients are unable to get a good night's sleep because of frequent episodes of upper airway obstruction. Apnea is most prevalent between the ages of 40 and 65 years and may affect at least 10% of men over age 40. Risk factors include obesity, craniofacial anomalies, acromegaly, and hypothyroidism. Although anatomic restriction of the upper airway can be observed in many patients, many patients with marginal upper airways do not experience obstruction during sleep, and severe sleep apnea commonly occurs in patients with apparently normal upper airways. This indicates that OSA is primarily a physiologic disturbance that may be exacerbated by anatomic factors.

Presentation

The classic "Pickwickian" patient has features described by Charles Dickens in *The Pickwick Papers:* obesity; a short, thick neck; a ruddy complexion; and a strong tendency to drop off to sleep. In most patients, the disorder is less obvious. Patients complain of headache and drowsiness or fatigue and may or may not volunteer a history of disturbed sleep. Some patients frequently awaken with shortness of breath or a sense of suffocation. Often, others in the household observe that the patient stops breathing during sleep. Many patients initially present with complaints of loud snoring and further workup reveals sleep apnea.

Diagnosis

Symptoms of hypersomnolence and loud snoring are highly suggestive of OSA. Findings on physical examination may or may not support the diagnosis, and a laboratory sleep study is indicated whenever there is significant clinical suspicion.

In many patients, the oropharyngeal airway appears constricted, owing to an elongated palate or uvula, tonsil hypertrophy, a large tongue, or redundant pharyngeal mucosa. Other common physical findings include a receding mandible or a shallow pharynx. However, some patients with OSA are thin and have no detectable upper airway anomaly.

Flexible endoscopy should be performed to evaluate the upper airway, at rest and during induction of negative pressure by Müller's maneuver. To perform this diagnostic trial, endoscopy is performed while the patient makes a deep inspiratory effort with the nose and mouth occluded. This maneuver should be performed while viewing the larynx and then repeated after repositioning to view the hypopharynx and then the velopharyngeal area. Collapse of the airway is estimated as a percent of the cross-sectional airway at each level. The pattern of collapse is considered to be of some value in predicting the success of surgical treatment, but the correlation is not absolute by any means.

Overnight polysomnography (sleep study) is required to establish the diagnosis of OSA and document severity. As patients sleep, electroencephalography is used to monitor the level of sleep and occurrence of dreams and arousals. Other monitored parameters include oxygen saturation, electrocardiaography, inspiratory muscle activity, and respiratory airflow. Apnea is defined as the cessation of respiratory airflow for at least 10 seconds. If inspiratory muscle activity continues, it is an obstructive apnea. Decreased respiratory volume constitutes hypopnea (Fig. 10–3). Some patients also have a significant number of nonobstructive central apneas. The average number of apneas per hour is the apnea index (AI), whereas the total number of respiratory disturbances per hour is the apnea–hypopnea index (AHI). An AI of > 5 is considered to be abnormal in the adult population; however, the level generally accepted as an indication for treatment is an AI ≥ 20. Other important indicators of severity are cardiac arrhythmias and oxygen saturation. In some patients, the severity of OSA varies from night to night; therefore, negative findings on only one sleep study do not necessarily rule out OSA.

Natural History

It is difficult to precisely assess the mortality of untreated OSA, because most people diagnosed with OSA are treated. However, an increased mortality rate has been reported for these patients. There are also increased risks of hypertension, cardiac arrhythmias, coronary artery disease, and cerebrovascular accidents, and it has been suggested that OSA plays a causal role in these disorders. Supporting this hypothesis is the association of blood pressure changes with apneic events. Blood pressure characteristically rises during apnea, reaching its peak when the patient arouses from sleep and the apnea is terminated. The magnitude of blood pressure elevation appears to correlate with the level of oxygen desaturation.

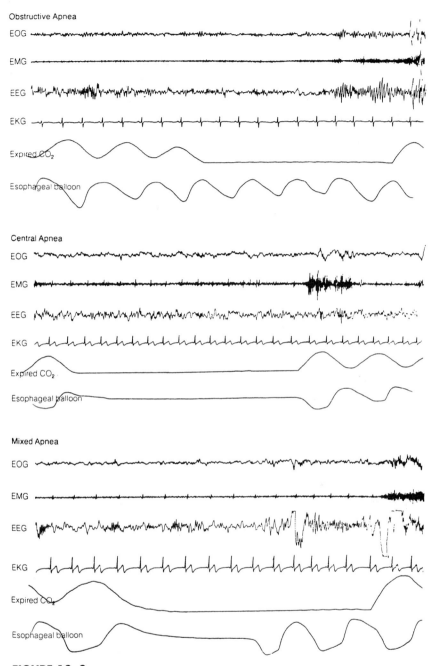

FIGURE 10-3
Apnea versus hypopnea. (From Hauri PJ. *Current Concepts: The Sleep Disorders*, Kalamazoo, MI: Upjohn, 1982.)

Treatment

In planning and assessing the results of treatment for OSA, it should be remembered that this is primarily a physiologic disturbance of upper airway control during sleep. Although anatomic restriction can exacerbate the problem, enlargement of the upper airway does not correct the fundamental derangement in control, and in many cases results in no clinical improvement.

The gold standard for treatment of obstructive sleep apnea is tracheotomy, which immediately bypasses the upper airway. One study, which supports the efficacy of tracheotomy, found that the mortality rate for patients whose OSA was treated conservatively was 11% but was 0% for those whose condition was managed by tracheotomy. The stoma can generally be occluded during waking hours so that speech is unimpaired. Nevertheless, the morbidity and social handicaps associated with tracheotomy are considerable. Tracheotomy sites require special care and may become infected. Patient with tracheotomies cannot protect their airway in water; hence, swimming is impossible and even bathing presents a risk. For these reasons, tracheotomy is generally indicated as primary management only for severe OSA. In patients with mild to moderate disease, other options are employed.

Obvious anatomic obstruction should usually be addressed before considering other treatment options. Tonsillectomy and/or adenoidectomy can be quite effective in some patients, particularly children. In contrast, relief of nasal obstruction, by removal of polyps or correction of deviation of the nasal septum, rarely has a profound impact on OSA.

Some conservative measures are frequently helpful in ameliorating OSA. Obese patients can substantially lessen the severity of OSA with weight loss. Sleep position is another factor that can be controlled. If apneas primarily occur in the supine position, then measures to promote sleeping on the side are helpful (such as sewing a tennis ball in the back of a pajama top). Alcohol and sedating medication should be avoided. There are no data to support the efficacy of many devices designed to pull the tongue anteriorly.

Nasal continuous positive airway pressure (CPAP) is extremely effective for most patients with OSA. The precise mechanism by which CPAP works is not known, but it has been shown to increase the volume and cross-sectional area of the pharynx. The effective pressure usually ranges from 7.5 to 12.5 cm H_2O and must be determined individually in the sleep laboratory for each patient. Nasal CPAP is most effective when used regularly, as symptoms recur when even one night is missed. Long-term use reduces the severity of OSA somewhat. Although CPAP is usually quite effective, some patients are noncompliant, or cannot tolerate the mask, often because of claustrophobia or nasal obstruction. Nasal surgery can usually relieve the obstruction, but for patients who are noncompliant because of other reasons, alternative management must be considered.

Uvulopalatopharyngoplasty (UP3) is usually the first-line surgical procedure for patients with OSA. This entails removal of the uvula and a portion of the soft palate, along with any palatine tonsil tissue that is present (Fig. 10–4). Usually very effective in eliminating snoring, UP3 is much less reliable in improving OSA. Success rates for UP3 in OSA patients range from 40% to 70%. Complications include

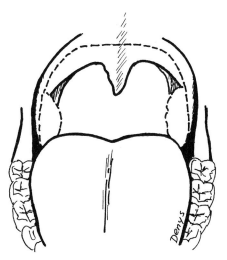 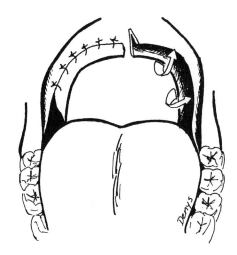

FIGURE 10–4
Uvulopalatopharyngoplasty.

palatal incompetence, with nasal reflux during swallowing, and naso-pharyngeal stenosis. These sequellae are uncommon, but when they occur, they are significant problems that are quite difficult to correct. A less severe complication is temporary decrease in taste function.

There are less invasive procedures for reducing the bulk of the palate, which are indicated primarily for snoring. These include laser-assisted uvulopalatoplasty and non–laser-assisted palatoplasty (using a bovie cautery). In both these procedures, small vertical cuts are made in the soft palate, on either side of the uvula (Fig. 10–5). As these lesions heal, the resultant scar tissue stiffens the palate. Often, one procedure is ineffective and repeat lesions must be created. An-

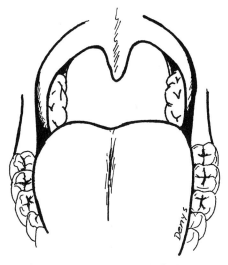 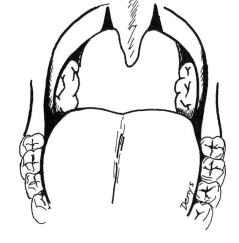

FIGURE 10–5
Laser-assisted uvulopalatoplasty.

other available option is radiofrequency ablation of the palate. All these approaches have documented efficacy for snoring and have been recommended by some for treatment of mild to moderate sleep apnea. However, there are no conclusive outcome data at present to support efficacy for sleep apnea.

For patients whose condition does not respond to UP3, there are other surgical options, depending on individual upper airway anatomy. A very large tongue base may be reduced by laser excision of a central trough or by radiofrequency ablation. A number of procedures have been devised to expand the hypopharynx: hyoid suspension pulls the hyoid bone upward and anteriorly using a suture or wire attached to the mandible, whereas mandibular advancement moves a segment of the anterior mandible forward, pulling with it the attached genioglossus muscle (Fig. 10–6). A less common and more invasive approach is surgical expansion of the maxilla.

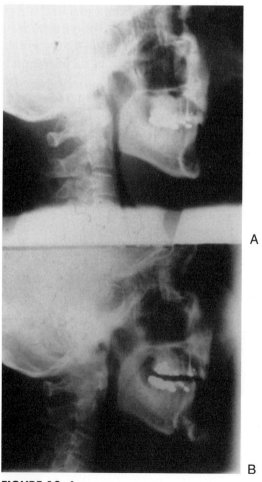

A

B

FIGURE 10–6
Mandibular advancement. Lateral skull films: **A,** before surgery; **B,** after advancement of a central segment of the mandible.

Any surgical procedure in a patient with OSA carries the increased risk of airway obstruction. Additionally, many patients have other medical conditions that increase surgical risks, including obesity, hypertension, and coronary artery disease.

When to Refer

Patients with signs and symptoms of OSA should undergo sleep studies. Home recording systems are useful for screening, but definitive diagnosis requires evaluation by a sleep laboratory. Otolaryngologic consultation is indicated to identify potentially correctable causes.

KEY POINTS

— Symptoms of hypersomnolence and loud snoring are highly suggestive of obstructive sleep apnea (OSA).

— Diagnosis of OSA requires polysomnography; however, negative findings on only one study do not rule out OSA.

— An apnea–hypopnea index of ≥ 20 is associated with increased mortality.

— Severe OSA should be managed by tracheotomy.

— Most patients with OSA respond to nasal continuous positive airway pressure.

— Uvulopalatopharyngoplasty is effective in only about 60% of patients with OSA.

Suggested Readings

Kryger MH. Management of obstructive sleep apnea. *Clin Chest Med* 13:481–492, 1992.

Maniglia AJ. Sleep apnea and snoring: an overview. *Ear Nose Throat J* 72:16–19, 1993.

Shepard JW. Hypertension, cardiac arrhythmias, myocardial infarction, and stroke in relation to obstructive sleep apnea. *Clin Chest Med* 13:437–438, 1992.

Functional Breathing Disorder

The vocal folds normally abduct with each inspiration. The term *paradoxical vocal fold motion* refers to inspiratory adduction of the vocal folds, narrowing the glottis and producing inspiratory stridor. Inspiratory adduction of the vocal folds sometimes occurs as result of neurologic disease, but more often, no organic cause is identified. The typical patient is a young woman, usually with an associated psychiatric condition, such as depression, obsessive-compulsive personality, adjustment reaction, borderline personality, passive-dependent personality, or somatization. The problem is assumed to be a functional breathing disorder, of psychogenic origin, such as a conversion reaction, or even malingering. Some studies have found a high incidence of sexual abuse during childhood of these patients. Many have a history of asthma, and in fact the episodes of laryngeal airway distress are often interpreted as asthmatic attacks. It has been suggested that these patients learn airway dysfunction as attention-seeking behavior. The episodes mimic the distress of asthma to a certain degree, but the major difference is that airway obstruction is during inspiration, whereas asthma is manifested by expiratory wheeze. It is a fairly easy task to restrict airflow during inspiration but nearly impossible to voluntarily produce expiratory wheeze.

A less common category of patients includes those with dysfunctional breathing during exercise. These patients are high-achieving athletes, in sports that involve extreme exertion and high oxygen demand, such as running. Stridor develops suddenly at peak exertion, typically at the end of a race. An organic cause is suspected in these patients, but the psychological profile is usually that of a compulsive achiever; the cause may be mixed. Some authors suspect either a neurogenic or structural impairment of the support of supraglottic structures.

Presentation

Patients present with recurring episodes of upper airway distress, often precipitated by anxiety or situational stress, or in the case of exercise-induced stridor, associated with extreme exertion. Many patients have a history of asthma, and in most cases, the episodes are often perceived as asthmatic attacks and treated as such. Patients with psychogenic or factitious breathing disorder will often experience some improvement with bronchodilator therapy, which perpetuates the notion that this is asthma. Ultimately, however, it is the failure to respond to medical management of asthma that suggests the diagnosis of functional breathing disorder.

Diagnosis

As just mentioned, the diagnosis is most often considered in patients whose condition does not respond to medical management. However, careful attention to the signs and symptoms will indicate that the episodes are not typical of asthma. Patients with functional breathing disorder have inspiratory stridor. Patients with asthma may develop inspiratory stridor during labored breathing, but the primary respiratory compromise is expiratory.

Physical examination during an episode of breathing distress is confirmatory. Auscultation of the chest rarely reveals significant wheezing. Flexible laryngoscopy reveals that the vocal folds actively adduct during inspiration. If stridor is severe, the resulting negative pressure in the upper airway sucks in pharyngeal and supraglottic mucosa. In some patients with exercise-induced dyspnea, supraglottic collapse is so severe that patients are considered to have a form of laryngomalacia.

A response to bronchodilator medication does not indicate that the problem is asthma. In fact, most patients' condition improves with nearly any treatment. A placebo injection of saline is often associated with a remarkable clinical improvement.

Natural History

The disorder is chronic and persisting but occasionally regresses spontaneously. Patients with psychogenic breathing disorder make multiple visits to the emergency department, where their condition always improves with treatment. The episodes of dyspnea, although frightening, are not life threatening.

Treatment

The first step in treatment is to reassure the patient that this is a known disorder and that it will not be fatal. It is often useful to show the patient videotape of the larynx during stridor, to provide some insight into the problem. Any irritative lesions of the larynx should be identified and treated. Over-the-counter cough suppressants are often helpful in reducing sensations of laryngeal irritation.

For patients with psychogenic issues, it is important to identify and treat associated psychiatric problems. Many will be resistant to treatment, but every effort should be made to have the patient seek evaluation from and advice by a psychiatrist. Patients with exercise-induced stridor may also have psychogenic issues to be addressed, usually related to the need to achieve, and many will benefit from psychiatric counseling.

The cornerstone of therapy for either patient group is breathing therapy by a speech pathologist, who will teach patients to control stridor. Patients are taught to focus on diaphragmatic breathing and keeping the upper airway open. Although this approach is usually effective, some patients' condition does not respond. In extreme cases, patients make such frequent trips to the emergency department that a tracheotomy may be indicated.

Some authors have recommended laryngeal surgery for selected patients with exercise-induced stridor. The goals are to prevent collapse of the supraglottic airway.

When to Refer

When the patient's condition does not respond to apparently adequate therapy for attacks of asthma, laryngeal breathing disorder should be suspected and evaluation by an otolaryngologist is indicated. Patients with attacks of inspiratory stridor should also see an otolaryngologist.

KEY POINTS

— Inappropriate adduction of the vocal folds causes inspiratory stridor.

— Most patients with laryngeal breathing disorder are initially given a diagnosis of asthma.

— The cause of the condition is usually psychogenic, such as a conversion reaction or malingering.

— Some patients have exercise-induced stridor.

— Breathing therapy should focus on diaphragmatic breathing, keeping the upper airway open, and breathing through the nose.

Suggested Readings

O'Connell MA, Sklarew PR, Goodman DL. Spectrum of presentation of paradoxical vocal cord motion in ambulatory patients. *Ann Allergy Asthma Immunol* 74:341–344, 1995.

Martin RJ, Blager FB, Gay ML, Wood RP. Paradoxical vocal motion in presumed asthmatics. *Semin Respir Med* 8:332–337, 1987.

Laryngospasm

Sudden and forceful closure of the larynx results in transient paroxysms of upper airway obstruction, with total occlusion or severe stridor. Laryngospasm is frightening but rarely fatal. With hypoxia, the laryngeal muscles relax, opening the airway. Laryngospasm is an exaggeration of the normal protective closure reflex. The most primitive function of the larynx is to prevent the entry of anything but air into the trachea. The larynx closes as part of swallowing and also closes in response to contact with foreign material. Laryngospasm most commonly occurs under light planes of general anesthesia, when reflexes are disinhibited. Less commonly, laryngospasm is episodic, recurrent, and not associated with anesthesia. In such patients, the stimulation threshold for laryngeal closure is lower and the response is sustained, owing to peripheral hypersensitivity and/or central disinhibition. Factors that have been implicated in this disorder include gastroesophageal reflux, inflammatory vocal fold lesions, viral neuropathy, focal dystonia, peripheral nerve injury, and seizure activity.

Presentation

Typically, each episode of laryngospasm is preceded by a sensation of irritation in the throat. This "tickle" or intense itching in the throat is followed by coughing or attempts to clear the throat and then either severe stridor or total airway occlusion. When total obstruction occurs, it is usually transient and does not result in loss of consciousness; however, the experience is usually quite frightening for the patient and bystanders.

Episodic laryngospasm in the ambulatory patient usually follows a viral illness or upper respiratory infection. Other patients note symptoms of gastroesophageal reflux. Much less commonly, spasms begin to occur several weeks following surgical trauma to a laryngeal nerve.

Diagnosis

The physician rarely observes actual episodes of obstruction but identifies the problem on the basis of the characteristic medical history and symptoms. It is important to establish that the event is actually obstruction and is not some other problem, such as dyspnea due to a pulmonary problem, or angina. The occurrence of inspiratory stridor is an important sign. It is also essential to establish the duration of episodes as objectively as possible. Laryngospasm is one of a very few disorders associated with upper airway obstruction of such rapid onset and dissipation. Psychogenic stridor and intermittent occlusion by a large polyp are the other possibilities. Obstruction that lasts several hours or days is more likely due to edema from an inflammatory process. Patients invariably overestimate the duration of obstruction, because events seem to "run in slow motion" during periods of extreme stress. A friend or family member who has observed the events can provide another perspective.

Physical examination between episodes of spasm usually reveals either a totally normal larynx or inflammatory evidence of gastroesophageal reflux. Much less frequently, vocal fold paralysis or weakness may be observed, indicating that the problem is due to a peripheral neuropathy, which may be of viral, surgical, or idiopathic origin. Occasionally a laryngeal lesion will be observed. A small laryngeal lesion may be responsible for stimulating the spasm, whereas a large pedunculated polyp may intermittently occlude the airway.

If gastroesophageal reflux is suspected, then a therapeutic trial of acid suppression is indicated. Twenty-four-hour pH monitoring may be considered as a diagnostic test. This is particularly helpful when an episode of laryngospasm is noted to coincide with a drop in pH. However, pH monitoring could be misleading. Reflux may be intermittent, without occurrence during the monitoring period. Furthermore, episodes of laryngospasm may not be temporally related to episodes of reflux. Instead, the inflammation of reflux may increase the sensitivity of mucosa, so that a variety of trivial stimuli could set off spasm. Another concern is that the monitoring catheter may precipitate spasm.

Very rarely, laryngospasm may be caused by an epileptic focus. If laryngospasm does not regress over time or respond to acid suppression, then electroencephalography should be performed.

Natural History

When episodic laryngospasm follows a viral illness, spasms generally become less frequent over time and usually resolve within 6 months. Spasm due to reflux may increase in severity and is far less likely to resolve spontaneously.

Treatment

Reassurance is a cornerstone of management of the disorder. Episodic laryngospasm is virtually never fatal and usually resolves with time. The frequency and severity of spasms can be reduced by avoiding laryngeal irritation and by taking cough suppressant medication, such as dextromethorphan. If gastroesophageal reflux is suspected, it should be treated with acid suppression. If an epileptic focus is identified, anticonvulsant medication is indicated.

Severe or persisting recurrences of laryngospasm may require more aggressive management. Injection of botulinum toxin into laryngeal muscle can reduce the severity of spasm. These injections must be repeated every few months. A permanent option is to resect a portion of the vocal fold to enlarge the airway.

When to Refer

Patients with acute episodes of upper airway obstruction should be examined by an otolaryngologist to rule out an anatomic cause.

KEY POINTS

— Sudden, severe upper airway compromise that comes on within seconds and dissipates quickly is due to laryngospasm.

— Recurrent episodes of laryngospasm may because by postviral neuropathy, gastroesophageal reflux, or laryngeal nerve injury.

— Recurrent laryngospasm is frightening but usually benign, and in most cases, it eventually resolves spontaneously.

— Medical management includes acid suppression, cough suppression, and occasionally, anticonvulsant medication.

— Rarely, botulinum toxin therapy or surgery is required to control spasms.

Suggested Readings

Loughlin CJ, Koufman JA. Paroxysmal laryngospasm secondary to gastroesophageal reflux. *Laryngoscope* 106:1502–1505, 1996.

Wani MK, Woodson GE. Paroxysmal laryngospasm after laryngeal nerve injury. *Laryngoscope* 109:694–697, 1999.

Laryngeal and Tracheal Stenosis

The segment of the airway formed by larynx and trachea has the narrowest cross-sectional area in the respiratory tract; therefore, even modest reduction of this lumen is poorly tolerated. Endotracheal intubation is the most common cause of laryngeal and tracheal stenosis. The underlying disease process is abnormal wound healing, with granulation tissue or scar contracture. Obstruction may be due to granulation tissue in the lumen, mucosal scar, or necrosis and collapse of the cartilage framework (Fig. 10–7). At the level of the larynx, scar tissue may immobilize the posterior ends of the vocal folds, preventing them from opening during inspiration (Fig. 10–8), or may form a web between the anterior vocal folds (Fig. 10–9). Posterior laryngeal scarring has a much greater impact on the airway than anterior scarring because the glottis is wider posteriorly. A significant anterior web often leaves a very adequate posterior airway (Fig. 10–9).

Intubation commonly results in minor mucosal trauma, such as edema or even abrasion, which heals uneventfully. The development of stenosis implies wound complication, a more serious injury, impaired healing, or a combination of these. Factors associated with an increased risk of stenosis include prolonged intubation, gastroesophageal reflux, and other medical illness, such as diabetes. Laryngeal stenosis is most frequent in patients who have a tracheotomy after prolonged intubation.

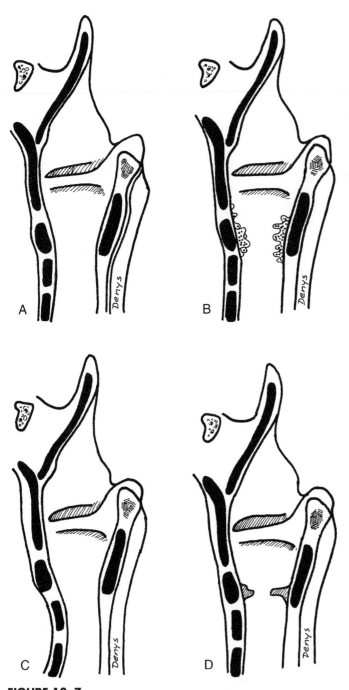

FIGURE 10-7
Mechanisms of tracheal stenosis: **A,** normal; **B,** intraluminal granulation tissue;
C, cartilaginous collapse; **D,** mucosal scar contracture.

Stenosis can also occur from scarring due to external trauma, inhalation injury, surgery, or radiotherapy. Gastroesophageal reflux has been implicated as a cause. Collagen vascular disease and amyloidosis can also affect the airway.

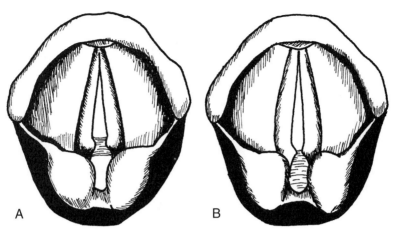

FIGURE 10-8
Laryngeal stenosis: **A,** scar band between vocal processes; **B,** posterior scar contracture.

Presentation

Symptoms of airway obstruction generally develop gradually. In some patients, stenosis develops, immediately after extubation; however, most patients do not have any unusual problems immediately after extubation, with airway symptoms developing months or even years

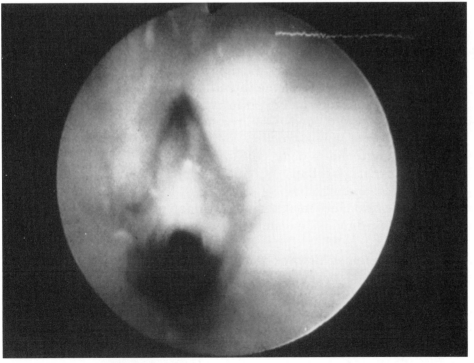

FIGURE 10-9
Endoscopic view of anterior glottic web.

212 - EAR, NOSE AND THROAT DISORDERS IN PRIMARY CARE

later. Sudden exacerbations are common. A typical patient first notices a gradual decrease in exercise tolerance or stridor with exertion. Patients present at varying points along the continuum of mild airway compromise to stridor at rest. A patient with partial obstruction is susceptible to acute exacerbations by temporary inflammatory processes, ranging from viral infections to allergic reactions. Therefore, it is not uncommon for a patient to have a series of acute episodes of obstruction, with relatively asymptomatic intervals. Some patients repeatedly present to the emergency department with episodes of airway obstruction. Because this edema often improves with medical therapy, patients are often assumed to have asthma.

Diagnosis

Stenosis should be considered in the differential diagnosis of any patient with respiratory compromise, particularly when there is a history of prior endotracheal intubation. Inspiratory stridor is the hallmark of upper airway obstruction. This may be audible or auscultation may be required for detection of stridor. Laryngeal stenosis and some cases of subglottic stenosis can be detected on physical examination, by mirror or office laryngoscopy. Tracheal stenosis and some cases of subglottic stenosis can be visualized only by bronchoscopy.

Spirometry is a very useful means of noninvasively assessing upper airway dysfunction. As discussed earlier in this chapter, upper airway obstruction preferentially impairs inspiratory airflow, whereas pulmonary disorders primarily affect expiratory flow. The flow–volume loop in a patient with stenosis of the larynx or extrathoracic trachea has a characteristic flattening of the inspiratory limb. Table 10–1 displays the airflow criteria for the diagnosis of extrathoracic airway obstruction. Obstruction of the intrathoracic portion of the trachea affects both inspiratory and expiratory airflow.

Imaging is essential to the diagnosis of laryngeal and tracheal stenosis, to localize the site of the obstruction, document the degree of airway compromise, and to aid in distinguishing between soft tissue in the lumen and cartilage collapse. Computed tomography is preferred because of the superior imaging of cartilage that it provides; however, magnetic resonance imaging is also valuable, particularly in constructing three-dimensional images of the airway (Fig. 10–10).

Definitive diagnosis of upper airway obstruction requires endoscopy. In patients with mild airway compromise, routine flexible bronchoscopy is usually reasonable. However, when the airway is marginal, endoscopy should be performed in the surgical suite, with the capability for airway management should this be necessary. Rigid bronchosopy provides airway control, allows precise quantification of the defect, permits endoscopic removal of granulation tissue, and may serve to temporarily dilate a stricture.

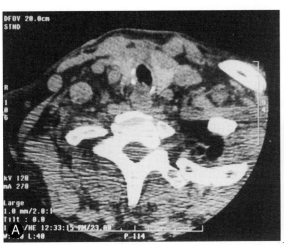
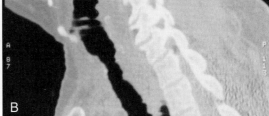

FIGURE 10-10
Tracheal stenosis: **A,** sagittal; **B,** axial.

Natural History

As mentioned above, postintubation stenosis may develop immediately following extubation or may develop gradually over months to years. Stenosis may stabilize, with a fixed level of impairment, or may continually progress. Frequent temporary exacerbations due to inflammatory processes can lead to progression of the underlying disease. Spontaneous remissions do not occur.

Treatment

The treatment of laryngeal and tracheal stenosis is either conservative and supportive, or surgical. Because surgical results are variable, many patients will choose to live with mild to moderate obstruction, particularly if they are poor surgery candidates owing to medical risks. Significant upper airway obstruction can usually be bypassed by tracheotomy, which may serve as definitive management or as a means of airway management during reconstruction. Granulation tissue can be excised endoscopically but often recurs. Subglottic stenosis is usually managed by laryngotracheoplasty, which uses a rigid graft to expand the cartilage framework (Fig. 10–11). Glottic stenosis is usually more difficult to treat because the optimal outcome, an adequate airway and normal voice, is often impossible to achieve. Unless normal motion can be restored to the vocal folds, the airway cannot be improved without impairing closure during phonation (Fig. 10–12). Tracheal stenosis is a special problem because the stricture is often below the level of a tracheotomy. The optimal treatment for tracheal stenosis is resection of the narrow segment and end-to-end anastomosis of the ends. This procedure is not possible if the involved segment is too long.

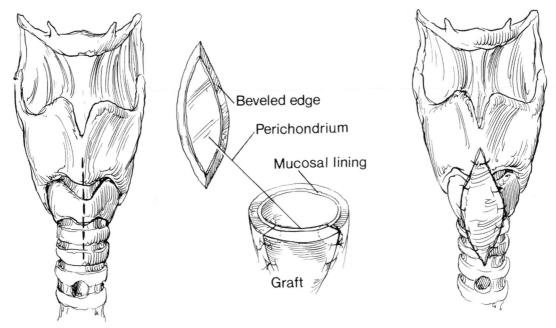

FIGURE 10–11
Laryngotracheoplasty. (From Alongo WA. Management of required larynageal stenosis. In Bailey BJ, Billor HF [eds.]: *Surgery of the Larynx*, Philadelphia: WB Saunders, 1985).

When to Refer

Patients with symptoms of chronic upper airway obstruction should be referred to an otolaryngologist for evaluation and possible surgical management.

When pulmonary function studies indicate upper airway obstruction, referral is indicated.

KEY POINTS

— Laryngeal or tracheal stenosis should always be considered in the differential diagnosis of breathing problems, particularly when there is a history of prior intubation.

— Inspiratory stridor is the characteristic physical sign of laryngeal and tracheal stenosis.

— Laryngeal stenosis can be recognized on office laryngoscopy.

— Spirometry is very useful in identifying and quantifying upper airway stenosis.

— Imaging is essential in detecting and characterizing subglottic and tracheal stenosis.

— Complete assessment of upper airway stenosis requires flexible bronchoscopy or rigid endoscopy.

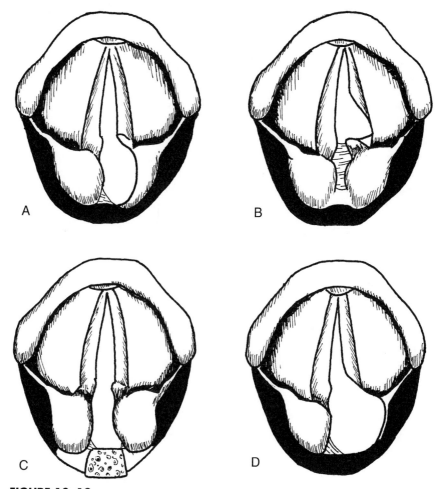

FIGURE 10–12
Treatment options for posterior laryngeal stenosis: **A,** medial arytenoidectomy; **B,** transverse cordotomy; **C,** posterior cricoid expansion graft; **D,** total arytenoidectomy.

Suggested Readings

Duncavage JA, Koriwchak MJ. Open surgical techniques for laryngotracheal stenosis. *Otolaryngol Clin North Am* 4:785–795, 1995.

Grillo HC, Donahue DM. Post intubation tracheal stenosis. *Semin Thorac Cardiovasc Surg* 8:370–380, 1996.

Other Neurogenic Causes of Upper Airway Obstruction

Regional dystonia (Meige's syndrome) consists of involuntary spasms of muscles in the face and neck, including blepharospasm, circumoral twitching, abnormal tongue and palate motions, and often significant laryngeal stridor.

Multiple system atrophy (also known as Shy–Drager syndrome) has been associated with laryngeal obstruction due to selective weakness or paralysis of the abductor muscles of the larynx. These patients develop progressive autonomic failure, with orthostatic hypotension.

Bilateral laryngeal paralysis is associated with varying degrees of airway distress. The voice is usually only moderately impaired because the vocal folds lie near the midline. The most common cause is surgical trauma during thyroidectomy. In such cases, airway distress may be immediate or may develop gradually as the vocal folds move toward the midline. Paralysis may also result from metastatic cancer. Current treatment is either a tracheotomy or a surgical procedure to widen the glottic airway, such as those used to treat glottic stenosis (Fig. 10–12). The former preserves vocal function, whereas the latter approach invariably impairs the voice to some degree.

Myasthenia gravis sometimes presents with upper aerodigestive tract symptoms, such as dysphagia and dysarthria. Rarely, patients present with airway obstruction due to laryngeal muscle weakness.

Swallowing

Disorders of swallowing are common, ranging from mild discomfort to life-threatening aspiration, or the complete inability to ingest anything. The prevalence of swallowing disorders is increasing with the aging of the population. It has been estimated that as may as 50% of elderly patients have some problems with eating, owing to such diverse factors as poor dentition, generalized weakness, dementia, and neuromuscular disease. Otolaryngologists are trained in evaluation of swallowing problems and have special expertise in the management of disorders of the pharyngeal phase of swallowing.

Management of swallowing disorders requires an understanding of normal processes and an appreciation of the many possibilities for dysfunction. This section reviews normal swallowing physiology, diagnostic approaches to dysphagia, and the management of the most frequent causes of pharyngeal dysphagia.

Physiology

Swallowing can be divided into three phases: oral, pharyngeal, and esophageal. The oral phase involves preparation of the bolus and transport into the pharynx. The pharyngeal phases involves transit of the bolus to the opening of the esophagus, which is a complex and highly coordinated act. During the third phase, ingested material passes through the esophagus and into the stomach.

The oral phase can be voluntarily controlled but is usually accomplished with little or no awareness. Solid foods must be chewed, whereas liquids require no special preparation prior to formation of the bolus. This is not a trivial task. If the bolus is not presented as a coherent mass, it is difficult for the pharynx to process it. Premature spillage into the pharynx or continued entry of material into the pharynx during or immediately after a swallow can lead to dangerous aspiration. The oral phase of swallowing may be impaired by diminished sensation, dental disease, or muscle weakness or incoordination. Sometimes tumors or tonsil hypertrophy can interfere with the oral phase.

The pharyngeal phase is not under conscious control; however, it is not a simple reflex. The process of getting the bolus into the esophagus, without aspiration through the larynx, is complex. Effective swallowing requires precise timing of motor activity and also considerable modification of timing and strength of muscle activity, based on sensory feedback about the size and consistency of the bolus. Incoordination, muscle weakness, decreased sensation, and mechanical obstruction can impair the pharyngeal phase.

The esophageal phase is less complex; its only goal is to propel food toward the stomach. Liquids can fall by gravity, but solids require propulsion by peristalsis. Inadequate propulsion or mechanical obstruction can impair the esophageal phase.

Diagnosis

When a patient complains of difficulty in swallowing, the first clinical task is to determine exactly what the patient is reporting (Table 10–2). Because swallowing is a complex activity, there are multiple ways for it to go awry. Food may "stick" or "go down the wrong way." Progressive difficulty in swallowing solid food usually indicates a mechanical obstruction, such as a tumor or stricture. Neurogenic dysphagia is usually worse with thin liquids, particularly in regard to aspiration. Pain can restrict intake when swallowing is otherwise normal. Finally, many patients who complain of difficulty in swallowing actually have a normal swallowing mechanism but have an ill-defined foreign-body sensation or the need to clear the throat (globus).

TABLE 10–2 • **KEY ELEMENTS OF HISTORY IN DYSPHAGIA**

Specific symptoms
    Obstruction
    Aspiration
    Nasal regurgitation
    Fatigue
    Pain
    Foreign-body sensation

Severity
    Weight loss
    Aspiration pneumonia
Onset, progression
Social history

When food "sticks," ask the patient to point to the area where the problem is perceived. Most patients with a mechanical obstruction can do this without hesitation. Another useful piece of information is the interval between onset of swallow and perception of the problem. Problems with the pharyngeal phase of swallow occur within 2 seconds, whereas esophageal dysfunction is manifested after 3 or 4 seconds, or as late as 20 seconds later.

How severe is the problem? Weight loss and/or aspiration pneumonia constitute the most compelling evidence of significant swallowing impairment. How long has the problem existed? New or progressive swallowing problems are more worrisome than chronic and persisting complaints.

Lifestyle and diet should be carefully covered in the history. For example, smoking and alcohol increase the risk of malignancy and bulimia can result in esophageal and pharyngeal inflammation.

Physical Examination. The physical examination should include a complete neurologic evaluation, with special attention to the fifth, seventh, ninth, tenth, twelfth cranial nerves. In particular, the examination should address lip competence, tongue strength, buccal control, and motion of the soft palate. The neck should be observed and palpated during swallow to assess laryngeal elevation and to detect any neck mass (including goiter). All mucosal surfaces in the upper aerodigestive tract should be inspected.

Diagnostic Tests. A barium swallow radiographic study demonstrates the lumen of the esophagus and detects intraluminal lesions, such as tumors or strictures, as well as compression by extrinsic masses, such as osteophytes or goiter. When pharyngeal dysfunction is suspected, a modified barium swallow should be performed. This requires collaboration between the radiologist and a speech pathologist. Instead of just swallowing liquid barium, the patient ingests small quantities of contrast substances of varying consistencies, ranging from very thin liquid to dry solids. Fluoroscopic images are carefully studied to evaluate motion, timing, and coordination and to detect possible residue or aspiration. It is important not only to identify residue or aspiration but also to identify the cause of the problem and possible corrective strategies.

Functional endoscopic evaluation of swallowing is essentially transnasal flexible endoscopic observation of the pharynx during swallowing. In actuality, it is impossible to see anything during a normal swallow, when the pharynx is completely collapsed. The examination can track motion of the bolus into the pharynx, and then detect any residue immediately after the swallow, particularly if the ingested material is colored. When the pharyngeal phase is abnormal, other dysfunction can be observed. For example, if there is delay in the initiation of the pharyngeal phase, material may be observed to enter the pharynx, without immediate reflex closure. The examination is most useful in patients who cannot be transported for radiographic studies. Scintigraphy uses a gamma counter to track a small amount of ingested radionuclide material. It provides accurate quantitative information about aspiration but does not demonstrate anatomy.

Esophagoscopy is the most specific means of identifying gastro-esophageal reflux disease (GERD), as well as infections and tumors of the esophagus. Esophageal manometry uses intraluminal pressure transducers to assess pressures and coordination during swallow. It is of limited usefulness in the evaluation of pharyngeal swallowing disorders, mainly documenting function of the upper esophageal sphincter.

Twenty-four-hour pH monitoring is a valuable test for detecting and quantifying acid reflux. It is also useful in establishing the temporal relationship of reflux and atypical symptoms, such as coughing and laryngospasm. The catheter is placed transnasally after the patient has fasted overnight. It is attached to a recording device, which permits the use of an event marker, so patients can accurately indicate the timing of symptoms. The most commonly used parameter of pH monitoring is the percentage of time that there is a pH < 4. The generally accepted norm is < 5%. The monitor can also differentiate reflux in the supine and recumbent positions and count the number of reflux events lasting more than 5 minutes, as well as the overall number of events. One drawback to pH monitoring is that reflux may be episodic (i.e., not every day). The sequellae of one significant episode of reflux can last for days.

Gastroesophageal Reflux

One of the most common causes of swallowing complaints is gastro-esophageal reflux, with inflammation and swelling of the pharyngeal and/or esophageal mucosa. In most cases, there is no objective evidence of a swallowing deficit. Unless inflammation is quite severe, patients do not have physical impairment of swallowing. Typically, patients complain of an abnormal sensation or pain during swallowing. Some may perceive that more effort is required to swallow, particularly for medication tablets or capsules. Between swallows, there is a sensation that "something is still there." The commonly used clinical term for this symptom complex is *globus hystericus.* The presumed mechanism for this is irritation of the pharynx and cricopharyngeus, with mucosal edema and/or reflex muscle spasm. Gastroesophageal reflux can also cause identifiable pathology of the esophagus, including esophagitis, webs, and strictures.

Diagnosis

A complaint of globus sensation strongly suggests the presence of GERD. Other symptoms of reflux include heartburn, water brash, and frequent belching. Some patients may experience symptoms of nocturnal reflux, such as frequent awakening with coughing, choking, or even fluid in the throat. However, even in patients who do not have these overt symptoms of reflux, gastroesophageal reflux is still the most common cause of globus symptoms.

Physical examination of the larynx and pharynx usually demonstrates erythema and edema, either diffuse or localized to the posterior larynx. Mucus stranding between the vocal folds is also common.

Esophageal pH monitoring is considered to be the gold standard for establishing the diagnosis of GERD. When findings are positive, such monitoring can be very helpful. However, reflux may be episodic and thus not detected if it does not occur during the monitoring period. A single episode of reflux can be responsible for symptoms that last for several days. Fluoroscopy with barium contrast is helpful for detecting webs, strictures, and spasms and occasionally may demonstrate active reflux. Manometry may reveal cricopharyngeal dysfunction, disordered esophageal paralysis, or esophageal achalasia.

The most cost-effective means of diagnosing reflux as a cause of dysphagia is a therapeutic trial of acid suppression. H_2 blockers, such as cimetidine or ranitidine, are effective in some but by no means all patients with GERD. Proton pump inhibitor medication—omiprazole or levamisole—has a much higher response rate. If there is no response to medical management of reflux within 4–6 weeks, then other diagnostic tests should be pursued.

Natural History

Gastroesophageal reflux disease is a chronic condition that often persists for years without progression. Although swallowing may be uncomfortable, oral intake is rarely affected. There is some evidence that GERD increases the risk of squamous carcinoma of the larynx, pharynx, or cervical esophagus; therefore, patients with GERD should be appropriately monitored.

Treatment

If there are no strictures or webs, medical management, consisting of acid suppression, dietary modifications, and lifestyle changes, is usually effective. Proton pump inhibitor medication is preferred over H_2 blockers because of its greater efficacy. Use of steroid medication and nonsteroidal anti-inflammatory drugs should be limited, because these drugs stimulate acid secretion. Spicy and acidic food should be avoided, and patients should not eat or drink for 1 or 2 hours before retiring. Smokers should give up tobacco. Obese patients should lose weight.

Resolution of symptoms may require 6–8 weeks. Acid suppression should be continued for at least 1 month after symptoms have disappeared, whereas recommended diet and lifestyle changes should be continued indefinitely. Many patients will require chronic acid suppression. Sometimes symptoms cannot be relieved, despite maximal medical therapy. In such cases, patients must usually learn to live with the symptoms. If persisting symptoms are sufficiently significant or if there is chronic inflammation of the larynx, gastric fundoplication should be considered. The morbidity of this procedure has been greatly reduced by development of the endoscopic approach.

Webs and mild to moderate strictures are generally managed by endoscopic dilation. Concomitant acid suppression and reflux management are usually indicated. Severe strictures respond poorly to endoscopic management. Surgical treatment requires total esophagectomy. A segmental resection is not possible because the esophagus lacks a serosa to ensure a watertight anastomosis. The resected esophagus is replaced by either a gastric pull-up or an intestinal graft. Either procedure is a major undertaking, with significant surgical morbidity and mortality.

When to Refer

Patients with presumably reflux-related dysphagia or globus after seemingly adequate medical therapy should be evaluated by a gastroenterologist. Otolaryngologic evaluation is also indicated, to detect and manage reflux-related changes in the larynx.

Webs or strictures may be managed endoscopically by a gastroenterologist, an otolaryngologist, or general surgeon. Patients with severe strictures or with significant GERD unresponsive to medical management should be evaluated by a surgeon and counseled regarding the possible need for surgery.

KEY POINTS

— Globus hystericus is a common symptom of gastroesophageal reflux disease (GERD).

— Patients with GERD may develop esophageal webs or strictures.

— Twenty-four-hour esophageal pH monitoring is considered to be the gold standard for documentation of acid reflux, but false negatives are possible when episodes are intermittent.

— If clinical signs and symptoms support the diagnosis of reflux, then a therapeutic trial of acid suppression is reasonable.

— Disease management should include lifestyle changes.

— Webs and mild to moderate strictures can usually be managed by endoscopic dilation.

— Recalcitrant reflux or severe stricture often requires surgery.

Suggested Readings

Henderson RD, Woolf C, Marryatt G. Pharyngoesophageal dysphagia and gastro-esophageal reflux. *Laryngoscope* 86:1531–1549, 1976.

Koufman JA. The otolaryngologic manifestations of gastroesophageal reflux. *Laryngoscope* 101(suppl 53): 1–78, 1991.

Zenker's Diverticulum

Zenker's diverticulum is a pulsion diverticulum that forms at the junction of the pharynx and esophagus. It is a lesion that occurs only in humans. Presumably the descent of the larynx during human development causes the circular fibers of the upper esophagus to follow an oblique course. The diverticulum forms in the region of the cricopharyngeal muscle, just above or below it, or even through the muscle fiber. It is presumed that cricopharyngeal dysfunction is involved in the pathogenesis of the diverticulum, because incomplete relaxation of this muscle leads to high intraluminal pressure.

Presentation

The classic symptom of a Zenker's diverticulum is regurgitation of undigested food, often several hours after eating. Most patients present after several years of progressive dysphagia. Other symptoms include choking on food, a gurgling sound in the neck, halitosis, coughing, and weight loss. The typical patient is older than 60 years and the ratio of men to women who have the disorder is 2:1.

Diagnosis

The symptoms of a patient with Zenker's diverticulum are usually sufficiently classic to strongly support a diagnosis. There are no characteristic physical findings. The pharynx and hypopharynx should be carefully inspected to rule out other pathology.

A barium swallow is the best means of demonstrating Zenker's diverticulum. (Fig. 10–13). The sac is distended by the barium, which remains in the sac after the esophagus is cleared. If food is present in the pouch, it may be apparent as defects in the barium. The barium swallow may also reveal distal pathology, such as webs or strictures in the esophagus, or a frank episode of gastroesophageal reflux.

Esophagoscopy is not necessary to diagnose Zenker's diverticulum but should be performed to determine the presence of other pathology. When the pouch is very large, the esophagoscope may preferentially pass into the pouch. This situation not only makes it difficult to examine the esophagus but also carries the risk of esophageal perforation.

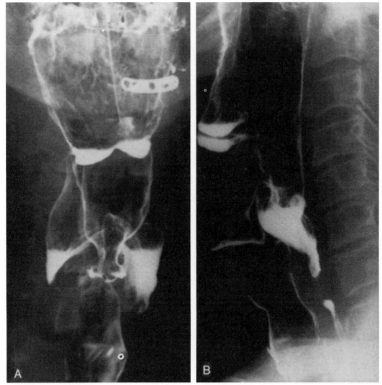

FIGURE 10-13
Zenker's diverticulum demonstrated with barium swallow (note pooling in vallecula):
A, anteroposterior; **B,** lateral. (From Stiernberg CM. Dysphagia and odynophagia. In
Meyerhoff WL, Rice DH [eds:] *Otolaryngology—Head and Neck Surgery,* Philadelphia:
WB Saunders, 1992).

Natural History

Patients develop progressive dysphagia. As the sac and its opening
enlarge, a greater proportion of food is diverted. This increases the
quantity of food available for regurgitation, and the risk of aspiration.
Additionally, a distended sac may externally compress the esophagus,
leading to mechanical obstruction. Progressive dysphagia leads to
nutritional impairment and cachexia. Rarely, squamous carcinoma
may develop in Zenker's diverticulum.

Treatment

No medical treatment is effective for Zenker's diverticulum; therefore,
surgical procedures are the only available therapeutic options. The
sac may be excised or suspended, or the party wall between the
sac and the esophagus can be divided. Each approach has its own
advantages and potential complications. Suspension of the sac carries
a lower risk of infection or fistula, because the esophagus is not incised.
However, this procedure does not eliminate the sac, and disruption

of the suspending suture or further inferior distension of the sac can result in recurrent symptoms. Both suspension and excision involve an external approach and potential damage to the recurrent laryngeal nerve. Excision may result in stricture if too much of the esophageal wall is removed with the sac. Endoscopic management is appealing because it avoids the morbidity of an external approach. However, for years many surgeons avoided endoscopic division of the party wall because they perceived it to carry a higher risk of leakage and possible mediastinitis. Endoscopic management has gained popularity in recent years because increasing experience has demonstrated its safety and technical advances have made it simpler. Better optics, fiberoptic lighting, and video capability have improved endoscopic visualization. An endoscopic stapling device may be used to simultaneously divide the wall and seal mucosal edges. The laser or electrocautery may also be used to divide the party wall.

No matter what procedure is used to deal with the sac, the cricopharyngeal muscle should also be divided, to reduce the risk of recurrence.

When to Refer

There is no effective medical management. Zenker's diverticulum can be treated only with surgery.

KEY POINTS

— Regurgitation of undigested food is the classic symptom of Zenker's diverticulum.

— Barium swallow is the best means of demonstrating Zenker's diverticulum.

— A low-residue diet may reduce sequellae, but definitive treatment requires surgery.

— Excision has been the treatment of choice for many years.

— Endoscopic management is gaining increasing acceptance.

Suggested Readings

Bonafede J, Lavertu P, Wood B, Eliachar I. Surgical outcome in 87 patients with Zenker's diverticulum. *Laryngoscope* 107:720–725, 1997.
Westrin KM, Ergus S, Carlsoo B. Zenker's diverticulum—a historical review and trends in therapy. *Acta Otolaryngol (Stockh)* 116:351–360, 1996.

Cricopharyngeal Achalasia

The cricopharyngeal muscle is a key component the upper esophageal sphincter. In a normal swallow, this muscle is relaxed at the end of the pharyngeal phase to allow the bolus to enter the esophagus. Inappropriate activity or fibrotic contracture of the cricopharyngeal muscle can significantly impede swallowing, sometimes leading to aspiration. Coordination of cricopharyngeal activity can be impaired by a number of neurologic disorders. Gastroesophageal reflux can lead to cricopharyngeal hyperactivity, but in some cases, no cause can be found for the abnormal function.

Presentation

Patients present with nonspecific difficulty in swallowing. Some patients may report choking on food.

Diagnosis

Cricopharyngeal dysfunction is demonstrated well by barium swallow (Fig. 10–14). The dysfunction may also be documented by manometry.

Treatment

Cricopharyngeal achalasia is usually treated by open surgical myotomy. Surgery is not indicated for mild problems, as there are significant surgical risks, including damage to the recurrent laryngeal nerve and fistula formation. Endoscopic dilation is ineffective. More re-

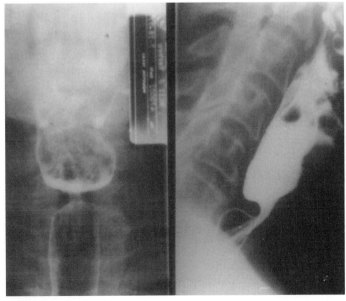

FIGURE 10–14
Cricopharyngeal achalasia demonstrated by barium swallow.

cently, endoscopic laser myotomy has been reported. Botulinum toxin injection of the muscle is another option that is sometimes effective; however, it requires repeat injection every few months and is of no benefit when the muscle is fibrotic. A trial injection is a good option, particularly if the patient is a poor surgical risk.

When to Refer

In a patient with dysphagia, when barium swallow demonstrates cricopharyngeal achalasia, surgical consultation is indicated.

KEY POINTS

— Spasm or fibrosis of the cricopharyngeal muscle impairs transit of food from the pharynx to the esophagus.

— Barium swallow clearly demonstrates cricopharyngeal achalasia.

— Botulinum injection may improve swallowing.

— Permanent treatment requires surgical myotomy.

Suggested Reading

Hellmans J, Pelemans W, Vantrappen G. Pharyngoesophageal swallowing disorders and the pharyngoesophageal sphincter. *Med Clin North Am* 65:1149–1171, 1981.

Neurogenic Dysphagia

Dysphagia is a complication of a variety of neurologic disorders, and in many, dysphagia may be the presenting symptom (Table 10–3).

TABLE 10–3 • **NEUROLOGIC DISEASES THAT IMPAIR SWALLOWING**

Stroke
Myasthenia gravis
Poliomyelitis
Muscular dystrophy
Inflammatory myopathy
Dementia
Amyotrophic lateral sclerosis
Parkinson's disease
Progressive supranuclear palsy
Multiple sclerosis
Head injury

Dysfunction may result from muscle weakness, sensory deficit, or central impairment.

Presentation

Neurogenic dysphagia presents with a broad spectrum of symptoms and severity. Various neurologic diseases can present with nearly identical swallowing problems. The clinical manifestations of dysphagia vary with the specific functional deficit, not the underlying neurologic disease. There are basically two types of swallowing problems—impairment of ingestion, and aspiration. Problems with ingestion can range from a sensation of "something in the throat" to inability to take in adequate nutrition to a complete inability to take in food or liquid. Sometimes ingested material refluxes out through the nose. If a patient cannot take in adequate nutrition, tube feedings can be used. This is inconvenient and socially restrictive. The second type of swallowing problem, aspiration, is a potentially life-threatening condition. Mild aspiration may result in coughing, with adequate clearing of aspirated material. However, severe aspiration, or "silent" aspiration that does not stimulate coughing, can cause aspiration pneumonia. Aspiration is a common mode of death in patients with chronic neurologic impairment.

Diagnosis

In most patients with neurogenic dysphagia, the swallowing problem is not the initial presentation of the disorder; there is already a clear medical diagnosis. This is particularly true for patients with head injury or stroke. But in some cases, dysphagia is the first clinical symptom. Detection of a neurogenic cause in such patients requires an awareness of the possible disorders and knowledge of their signs and symptoms.

Associated signs of upper aerodigestive tract dysfunction, such as hoarseness or dysarthria often accompany neurogenic dysphagia. There may be obvious symptoms of generalized neurologic disease, such as limb weakness, tremor, or sensory deficits. Patients with myasthenia gravis note that symptoms are worse later in the day or evening, owing to fatigue.

A careful neurologic evaluation is always indicated in the workup of dysphagia. If neurogenic disease is suspected, neurologic consultation is indicated.

Modified barium swallow is particularly important in the evaluation of patients with possible neurogenic dysphagia. Modified barium swallow helps to characterize the specific functional defect, aids in planning rehabilitative therapy, and identifies dangerous aspiration.

Natural History

The underlying disease process dictates the natural history of the disorder. For example, a patient with a stroke will have a sudden catastrophic lesion that may remain stationary or gradually improve. A patient with amyotrophic lateral sclerosis (ALS) will have inexorable progression of disease.

Treatment

This chapter will not deal with the medical management of the underlying neurologic disorder. However, it is clear that the management of neurogenic dysphagia begins with the medical therapy of any treatable disease process. For example, patients with myasthenia gravis should have maximal medical therapy for that disorder and swallowing therapy plays a supportive role.

In most patients with neurogenic dysphagia, the lesion resulting in swallowing dysfunction is irreversible, as after a stroke, or even progressive, as in ALS. Treatment is based on the specific functional defects responsible for the swallowing problem and the likelihood for recovery or progression.

Swallowing therapy includes modification of food consistency, controlling posture during swallowing, exercise programs designed to strengthen swallowing muscles, and instruction in safe swallowing techniques. In patients with aspiration, thicker liquids are less likely to spill into the airway, whereas in patients with poor transport, solid food is poorly tolerated, and thin liquids are ingested more easily. Examples of postural changes include (1) sitting up straight and slightly forward and (2) turning the head to close of the paretic side of the pharynx or larynx.

Surgical Treatment

Nasopharyngeal regurgitation results from weakness of the palate. If the problem is a fixed unilateral paralysis or paresis, then a palatal adhesion procedure can be performed to close off the velopharyngeal port on the affected side. If the weakness is bilateral or due to a progressive problem, such ALS, then surgery is inappropriate. Some patients may benefit from a palate lift prosthesis.

The role of cricopharyngeal myotomy in patients with neurogenic dysphagia is controversial. The procedure may be helpful in cases with uncoordinated swallow, fibrosis of the cricopharyngeus, or when constrictor muscles are weakened, so that there is inadequate force to propel the bolus through the upper esophageal sphincter. However, the opening of the upper esophageal sphincter requires elevation and anterior displacement of the larynx, and if this is impaired, myotomy will not improve swallowing. It is difficult to predict a priori which patients will benefit. Injection of botulinum toxin into the cricopharyngeus has been suggested as a means to predict the results of myotomy, but there may be no correlation of effect. Weakening the muscle is not the same as surgically transecting it, particularly if the muscle is fibrotic. In selecting patients, for myotomy, it is important to weigh the likelihood of benefit versus the risks of surgery for each individual patient.

Vocal fold medialization is indicated for treatment of aspiration in patients with laryngeal paralysis. Paralysis alone does not result in aspiration, unless the glottic gap is extremely wide. However, other problems, such as pharyngeal weakness or sensory deficit, can impair the ability to compensate. In most patients with laryngeal paralysis who aspirate, medialization procedures such as Teflon injection or thryoplasty are inadequate, and arytenoid adduction is required.

In patients with severe aspiration, it may be necessary to surgically separate the airway and digestive tract. In all such procedures, a tracheotomy is required and vocal function must be sacrificed.

When to Refer

Neurogenic dysphagia is best managed by a dysphagia management team, including an otolaryngologist, a speech pathologist, and often a gastroenterologist.

KEY POINTS

— Many neurologic diseases impair swallowing.

— Neurogenic dysphagia causes two broad categories of problems: limitation of ingestion and aspiration.

— Aspiration pneumonia is the most serious complication of neurogenic dysphagia.

— Swallowing therapy can help patients improve intake and sometimes decrease aspiration.

— Several surgical procedures can be used to improve swallowing in selected patients.

— In patients with severe aspiration, the airway should be surgically separated from the aerodigestive tract.

Suggested Readings

Eisle DW, Yarington CT, Lindeman RC, et al. The tracheoesophageal diversion and laryngotracheal separation procedures for treatment of intractable aspiration. *Am J Surg* 157:230–236, 1989.

Logemann JA. The role of the speech language pathologist in the management of dysphagia. *Otolaryngol Clin North Am* 21:637–648, 1988.

11

NECK MASSES

• Steven Long, M.D.

INTRODUCTION

A lump in the neck is a disturbing clinical finding. It potentially indicates a severe problem, and the differential diagnosis is broad. The diversity of problems that can manifest as a neck mass is directly related to the anatomic complexity of this region. The neck serves dual roles as a flexible support structure and a conduit for connections between the head and body. Consequently, components of the nervous, gastrointestinal, respiratory, cardiovascular, and lymphatic systems are compressed within a relatively small cross-sectional area. The most common neck mass is a lymph node that has been enlarged by infection or tumor. Less commonly, lymph nodes are enlarged by drug reaction or by idiopathic inflammatory diseases, such as sarcoidosis. Congenital anomalies of the neck are common, owing to the complex embryologic development of the region. A neck mass may also be a primary tumor. This chapter presents a strategy for the initial approach to diagnosis and then covers the management of the most common neck masses.

Diagnosis

The probability ranking of items in the differential diagnosis of a neck mass varies profoundly with the age of the patient. A neck mass in a newborn is by definition a congenital lesion. Congenital neck anomalies also commonly present throughout childhood and young adulthood, but the majority of neck masses in children and young adults are of infectious origin. The likelihood of tumor increases with age. In a patient older than 40 years of age, a neck mass should be assumed to be a malignancy until proven otherwise.

The first step in the medical history is to differentiate between acute and more indolent processes (Table 11–1). As a rule, rapid growth and pain indicate infection—in a lymph node or in a congenital cyst—whereas a slowly growing mass raises the suspicion of malignancy. There are exceptions, however. Some tumors can grow rapidly, and a granulomatous infection may grow slowly, with little or no pain. The history should also investigate potential exposure to specific infections, such as tuberculosis in a family member, recent acquisition of a new pet, or travel to a foreign country. Patients who present with infection in a congenital cyst may give a history of previous similar occurrences. Systemic signs, such as fever, malaise, and cachexia, may serve as indicators as to the nature of the pathology.

A key component of the physical examination is careful inspection and palpation of the neck. The location, attachments, and consistency of the mass provide valuable cues. Size is also important, as a mass >2 cm in diameter is more likely to be a malignant tumor. The physical

---

TABLE 11–1 • **COMMON NECK MASSES**

Inflammatory
    Acute
        Viral
        Bacterial
    Chronic
        Nontuberculous
        Tuberculous
        Cat scratch
Congenital
    Cystic
        Thyroglossal duct cyst
        Dermoid
        Branchial cleft cyst
    Vascular
        Hemangioma
        Cystic hygroma
    Congenital torticollis
Neoplastic
    Metastatic
    Lymphoma
    Thyroid tumor

examination should also include inspection of all mucosal surfaces of the mouth and pharynx, and otoscopic examination. It is important to seek potential infection or tumor in regions drained by the cervical lymphatics. Fluid in the middle ear of an adult should be regarded as a potentially ominous sign of a nasopharyngeal tumor.

Hematologic studies are often informative. The white blood cell count is usually elevated in acute infectious processes, and examination of the peripheral blood smear may reveal atypical lymphocytes in patients with infectious mononucleosis. Laboratory studies are also very important when there is a clinical suspicion of acquired immunodeficiency syndrome (AIDS).

Plain films of the neck are not useful in the evaluation of neck masses. However, a chest x-ray is usually indicated because it is important to seek possible infection or tumor in the lungs. Other types of imaging are sometimes needed to resolve specific issues. For example, ultrasound is useful in differentiating cystic and solid lesions. Computed tomography (CT) is an excellent technique for imaging the structures of the neck, particularly when performed with infusion of contrast. It can delineate a cyst from a solid tumor, establish location with respect to other structures (e.g., the carotid artery, the thyroid gland), and indicate vascularity. However, imaging is not indicated in most cases; it should be used only to answer specific clinical questions.

Fine-needle aspiration (FNA) is an extremely valuable tool for the evaluation of neck masses when a tumor is suspected. A small-bore (22-gauge) needle is used to aspirate tissue fragments (Fig. 11–1). The

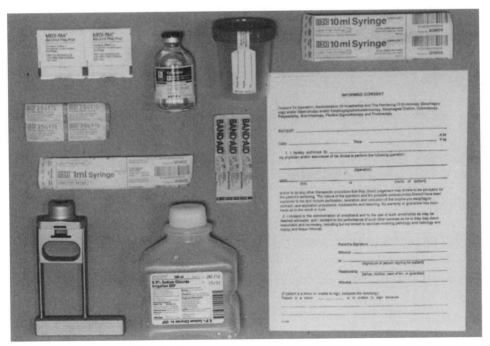

FIGURE 11–1
Equipment for performing fine-needle aspiration biopsy.

234 – EAR, NOSE AND THROAT DISORDERS IN PRIMARY CARE

needle contents are placed on a slide, then processed and stained for microscopic cytologic examination, much like a pap smear. Fine-needle aspiration is rapid, inexpensive, and simple to perform. Several studies have indicated an accuracy >90% in the diagnosis of head and neck masses. Fine-needle aspiration can also be helpful in eluci-dating the cause of infection or for aspirating pus when an abscess has formed.

A therapeutic trial of antibiotics or antituberculous medication is often helpful in confirming the diagnosis.

Open biopsy is reserved for those cases in which the diagnosis remains elusive or when the FNA indicates a neoplasm requiring histologic evaluation, such as a lymphoma. If the mass is suspected to be metastatic cancer, it should not be excised until after a thorough search for a primary tumor.

KEY POINTS

— A neck mass in a child or young adult is more likely to be inflammatory, whereas tumors are more common in older adults.

— The diagnosis is frequently established by findings on the medical history and physical examination.

— Fine-needle aspiration is an extremely useful tool in the evaluation of neck masses.

— Open biopsy should not be undertaken unless a thorough evaluation has failed to establish the diagnosis.

Suggested Reading

Olto RA, Bowes AK. Neck masses: benign or malignant? Sorting out the causes by age group. *Postgrad Med* 88:199–204, 1990.

Inflammatory Lymphadenopathy

Acute Lymphadenitis

A painful and swollen neck mass is most often an infected lymph node. Benign palpable lymph nodes are common in healthy children—in the neck or axillary or inguinal regions. Such nodes are usually <1 cm in diameter, soft, nontender, and eventually resolve spontaneously. Most children with enlarged lymph nodes never present to a physician for this complaint. In adults, benign lymphadenopathy is less com-mon. *Lymph nodes become worrisome when they are tender or >1 cm in diameter.*

Presentation. Viral infection of the pharynx and/or upper respiratory tract is an extremely common cause of cervical lymphadenopathy. The clinical course is generally benign and self-limited and rarely requires intervention. Impressive lymphadenopathy is often encountered in infectious mononucleosis, caused by the Epstein–Barr virus (EBV). These patients typically present with malaise, fever, anorexia, throat pain, and rapidly enlarging neck nodes. Occasionally, the lymphadenopathy is dominant presenting complaint.

The peak occurrence of bacterial lymphadenitis is between the ages of 1 and 5 years. Usually the submandibular or deep upper jugular nodes are involved and the most common organisms are group A β-hemolytic *Streptococcus* or *Staphylococcus.* The overlying skin is erythematous and tender. The patient usually presents after several days of an upper respiratory infection (URI) with a gradually enlarging neck mass. The adenitis may be secondary to an infection in the head and neck region, such as otitis media or tonsillitis. However, the source of the infection is usually not apparent.

Diagnosis. Acute lymphadenitis is diagnosed on the basis of a history of the sudden appearance of a painful neck mass and the physical findings of a tender, firm, mobile mass. However, the history and physical findings frequently fail to differentiate viral from bacterial infections. Both types of infection may present with either single or multiple enlarged nodes. Bacterial lymphadenitis is generally associated with more local reaction than viral adenitis, including tenderness as well as erythema and edema of the overlying skin.

In bacterial adenitis, the physical examination should carefully search for a primary infection, such as otitis, tonsillitis, or a dental or scalp abscess. The location of the lymphatic infection offers clues to the location of a primary infection, as lymph node groups drain specific anatomic areas (Fig. 11–2, Table 11–2). However, the primary source is often not found.

A peripheral blood smear may be helpful in distinguishing viral from bacterial infection and is particularly informative in patients with infectious mononucleosis. The diagnosis of infectious mononucleosis is confirmed by specific hetrophile antibody titers, EBV culture, or monospot or heterophile test.

As a rule, soft tissue neck mass, plain films do not demonstrate any pathologic findings in patients with cervical lymphadenitis. Computed tomography or magnetic resonance imaging (MRI) can precisely delineate the mass and surrounding normal structures, but such information is not necessary for the management of uncomplicated lymphadenitis. Imaging is indicated when the mass is very large, when the diagnosis is not clear, when there is airway obstruction, or when suppuration and abscess formation are suspected.

Natural History. In most viral illnesses, lymphadenopathy will resolve within 5–10 days. Adenopathy may persist for 2 weeks in

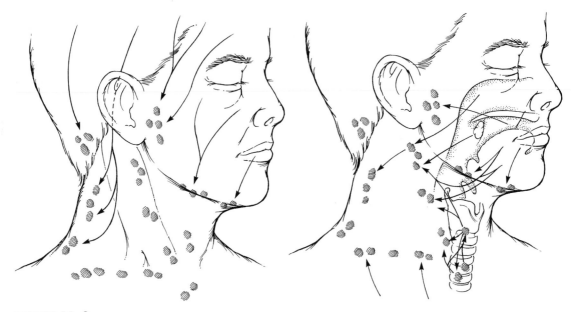

FIGURE 11–2
Cervical lymph node groups: external (*left*) and internal (*right*) drainage. Arrows indicate drainage pathways. (From McGuirt WF Sr. Differential diagnosis of neck masses. In Cummings CW, et al [eds]: *Otolaryngology—Head and Neck Surgery*, 3rd ed., St. Louis: Mosby, 1998.)

cases of chickenpox, mumps, herpes, and measles, and for up to 6 weeks in patients with infectious mononucleosis.

Bacterial lymphadenitis may undergo central necrosis and become fluctuant. A small, unilocular abscess occasionally resolves without drainage or any treatment. It may also rupture and drain, resulting in either healing or a chronically draining fistula. Advanced cervical adenitis may cause airway compromise or dysphagia. The infection may spread to surrounding tissues, resulting in cellulitis or a deep neck abscess. Deep neck infections have the potential for severe complications, including jugular venous thrombosis or mediastinitis.

Treatment. All patients with cervical adenitis should be treated with antibiotics. Although viral lymphadenitis actually requires only

TABLE 11–2 • **PATTERNS OF CERVICAL LYMPHATIC DRAINAGE**

Node Group	Area Drained
Preauricular	Eyelids, external ear, lateral scalp
Submental	Anterior tongue, mouth, lower lip
Submandibular	Teeth, gums, tongue, central face
Jugulodigastric	Tonsils, tongue, pharynx
Upper deep cervical	Tonsils, tongue, pharynx
Lower deep cervical	Posterior scalp and neck

supportive care, it is not possible to be certain in any patient that a bacterial infection is not involved. Therefore, for practical purposes, all patients with acutely swollen lymph nodes should be assumed to have a bacterial infection. The initial treatment for uncomplicated acute lymphadenitis is a 10-day course of oral antibiotic therapy with a β-lactamase–resistant antibiotic, covering for the most likely organisms, *Staphylococcus* and *Streptococcus*. If there is no improvement within 2 days, fine-needle aspiration (FNA) should be performed to seek and drain any pus and to obtain specimens for culture and sensitivity testing.

Intravenous antibiotics are indicated if the infection does not improve on oral medication or when the patient presents at a more advanced stage of disease. A large mass, significant surrounding cellulitis, airway compromise, and signs of septicemia are all indications for intravenous antibiotics.

Surgical excision of acutely infected nodes is not often indicated. The infection nearly always responds to antibiotic therapy. In addition, local inflammation greatly increases the surgical risks of bleeding and damage to nerves or vessels. However, drainage is indicated if adenitis progresses to abscess formation, to hasten resolution and reduce the risk of progression to a more serious infection. Small abscesses may respond to needle aspiration, whereas large abscess and those with significant surrounding cellulitis usually require incision and drainage. Surgical excision should be considered when the infection fails to respond to an adequate trial of antibiotics and when results of FNA fail to establish a diagnosis.

When to Refer. Consultation is indicated when lymphadenitis does not respond to antibiotics, when the mass is impinging on the airway, or when suppuration develops and drainage is contemplated.

KEY POINTS

— Peak occurrence of acute lymphadenitis is between the ages of 1 and 5 years.

— It is difficult to differentiate viral and bacterial lymphadenitis.

— Antibiotic therapy is indicated for all patients.

— If empiric antibiotic therapy fails, fine-needle aspiration should be performed for culture and sensitivity.

— In general, acutely inflamed lymph nodes should not be excised.

— Suppurated nodes should be drained by needle or incision.

Suggested Readings

Chesney PJ. Cervical adenopathy. *Pediatr Rev* 15:276–284, 1994.

Herzog LW. Prevalence of lymphadeopathy of the head and neck in infants and children. *Clin Pediatr* 22:485–487, 1983.

Swartz MN. Lymphadenitis and lymphangitis. In: Mandell GL, Bennett JE, Dolin R eds.: *Principles and Practice of Infectious Diseases,* 4th ed., vol. 1. New York: Churchill Livingstone, 1995, pp 936–944.

Chronic Cervical Lymphadenitis

A number of infectious agents can cause indolent infection of lymph nodes in the neck. Most common among such infections are nontuberculous mycobacterial adenitis, tuberculosis (TB), and cat-scratch disease. Less common infections include toxoplasmosis, actinomycosis, tularemia, histoplasmosis, brucellosis, and cytomegalovirus.

Nontuberculous mycobacteria (NTM) are found in water, soil, and dust. Infection by these organisms predominantly occurs in children between the ages of 1 and 5 years. Because nontuberculous lymphadenitis is not observed in children too young to put foreign objects into their mouths or in those old enough to know better, it is presumed that the infection is acquired through intraoral contact. The most common pathogenic NTM species is *Mycobacerium avium-intracellulare.* An association has been noted between NTM adenitis and the practice of using a lower temperature in the hot water tank. A lower hot water heater temperature has been advocated to avoid scalding injuries, but the lower temperature permits the overgrowth of NTM in the water heater.

Tuberculous cervical adenitis is uncommon in the United States but is quite common in many developing countries, where it may be responsible for as much as 45% of cervical adenopathy. In the United States, tuberculous lymph node infection is usually associated foreign travel, previous tuberculosis, or immunodeficiency. Cervical adenopathy is not a usual clinical feature of tuberculosis. Only approximately 5% of patients with tuberculosis infection have cervical adenopathy. By contrast, active pulmonary disease is present in only 5% of patients with cervical tuberculosis.

Cat-scratch disease is an indolent lymphatic infection caused by *Rochalimaea henselae.* It is most frequently associated with exposure to a cat, or, more rarely, a dog; however, there is frequently no history of pet exposure. The yearly incidence of cat-scratch disease is between 1.8 and 9.3 cases per 100,000 people. Most cases occur between September and January.

Presentation. The clinical presentation of chronic lymphadenitis is variable but is generally more indolent than that of an acute bacterial adenitis. Some patients do not present until the mass has been present for 1 or 2 months. Masses may be single or multiple but are usually unilateral. There are subtle differences in presentation among type of adenitis, but these differences are not sufficiently constant or clear-cut to be firm clinical indicators.

Tuberculous nodes generally present in the posterior triangle, whereas nontuberculous mycobacterial adenitis and cat-scratch disease usually occur in the submandibular or high jugular region. Tuberculous nodes are usually firm and nontender, whereas many patients with cat-scratch disease present with malaise, fever, and tenderness of the overlying skin. In just under 50% of patients with cat-scratch disease, the inoculation site is clinically apparent. Approximately 10% of cat-scratch masses are fluctuant.

Diagnosis. Differential diagnosis often difficult, as the clinical presentations of these infections are similar and the final results of mycobacterial cultures are not available for weeks. Unfortunately, optimal management is different for each of the three most common types of chronic lymphadenitis and therefore precise identification of the pathogen is crucial (Table 11–3). It is particularly important to distinguish between tuberculous and nontuberculous mycobacterial infections, as the former is best managed by medication and requires screening of contacts, whereas the latter can be managed only by surgery. A chest radiograph should be performed to look for evidence of pulmonary tuberculosis, even though most patients with cervical tuberculosis do not have pulmonary involvement. Skin and serologic tests are often helpful in differentiating these patients.

Results of skin testing with purified protein derivative should be positive in patients with tuberculous lymphadenitis, borderline (<15 mm induration) in those with nontuberculous mycobacterial infection, and negative in patients with cat-scratch disease. Recently, a serologic test has become available for *R. henselae,* the causative organism for cat-scratch disease, and this test has a 90% positive predictive value.

Interpretation of skin test results is complicated by the fact that a patient who has a neck mass caused by something other than TB could have positive skin test results because of previous exposure. Further, skin test results may be falsely negative in patients who are anergic or immunodeficient. Therefore, fine-needle aspiration (FNA) should be performed to confirm the diagnosis. Cytologic examination may reveal granulomatous inflammation in tuberculous or nontuberculous nodes or the cat-scratch bacillus. Acid-fast organisms are rarely

TABLE 11–3 • DIAGNOSIS OF CHRONIC LYMPHADENITIS

	Tuberculous	Nontuberculous	Cat-Scratch
Chest x-ray	±	Negative	Negative
Purified protein derivative	Positive	Borderline	Negative
Rh serology	Negative	Negative	Positive
Fine-needle aspiration	Granuloma	Granuloma	±Bacillus

seen, either on FNA or biopsy, except in patients with AIDS. Fine-needle aspiration should also be used to obtain culture specimens. Occasionally, FNA is useful in demonstrating other less common pathogens, such as fungi.

Biopsy of a tuberculous node may result in a chronically draining fistula. Therefore, biopsy should be deferred as long as a tuberculous infection is suspected. A therapeutic trial of antituberculous medication is a reasonable approach. If there is no response to such medication, then excisional biopsy is indicated. Biopsy of tuberculous and nontuberculous nodes demonstrates caseating granulomas and sometimes acid-fast organisms. Histologic signs of cat-scratch disease include lymphoid hyperlasia, proliferation of arterioles, reticulum cell hypertrophy, and, in more advanced cases, scattered granulomata. The Warthin–Starry silver stain is used to detect the cat-scratch bacillus.

Natural History. When left untreated, both tuberculous and nontuberculous nodes will gradually enlarge and suppurate, resulting in chronically draining sinus tracts.

Tuberculosis is a chronic, systemic illness, and the disease may reactivate years after seemingly adequate drug therapy. Stress and steroid therapy can both contribute to reactivation. Nontuberculous infection may lie dormant in adjacent tissue after seemingly adequate gross resection of disease, and clinical infection has been reported to recur up to 7 years after apparent resolution.

By contrast, cat-scratch disease is almost always a self-limited infection. Nearly all cat-scratch lesions eventually resolve, but the process may take weeks or months. In a small percentage of patients, the infection is severe and systemic, with such complications as encephalitis, pneumonia, and hepatitis.

Treatment. As mentioned above, treatment is different for each of the etiologic agents.

Tuberculosis of the cervical lymph nodes is best managed by medication. Surgical intervention may result in a chronically draining fistula. Therefore, surgical intervention is indicated only when there is no response to medication.

Nontuberculous mycobacteria are resistant to antituberculous medication. Therefore, cervical lymph nodes infected by NTM should be treated by surgical excision. Incision and drainage of either tuberculous or nontuberculous nodes is contraindicated, as this will often result in a chronic draining fistula. When the infection involves multiple nodes near important structures, such as the facial nerve, curettage has been recommended, to achieve maximal removal of infected tissue without creating deformity or handicap.

Cat-scratch disease is usually a self-limited but somewhat protracted disease. Lesions almost always eventually resolve without specific treatment. No antibiotic therapy has been demonstrated to be effective. Surgery is not required, but if the diagnosis cannot be established by FNA or serologic testing, then excisional biopsy is generally curative as well as diagnostic.

Other Causes of Cervical Adenitis

When a causative organism is not identified for persisting lymphadenitis, an excisional biopsy should be performed and used to rule out neoplasm and guide treatment. Occasionally an unusual organism will be identified, such as actinomycosis, histoplasmosis, or CMV (Table 11–4).

Toxoplasmosis results in infection by the parasite *toxoplasma gondii,* acquired by ingestion of poorly cooked meat or of oocytes excreted in cat feces. In immunocompetent patients, the disease is mild or asymptomatic, resolves spontaneously, and is best diagnosed by serologic testing. In patients with AIDS, the disease may result in fatal disease of the central nervous system (CNS), and false-negative serology makes diagnosis difficult. Combination therapy with pyrimethamine and sulfonamides has some efficacy in this disease.

Tularemia is another cause of acute lymphadenopathy, usually accompanied by fever, tonsillitis, painful lymph nodes, ulcers, chills, fatigue, and headache. It is transmitted to humans by rabbits, ticks, and contaminated drinking water. It occurs in the West and South in the United States. The diagnosis is based on serology and culture, and the disease usually responds to erythromycin.

Bubonic plague is very rare in the United States, but occasional outbreaks occur in the western United States. Fleas and rodents, especially prairie dogs, carry the causative organism, *Yersinia pestis.* The disease is characterized by necrotic draining nodes, referred to as buboes. Diagnosis is made on the basis of Gram's stain and culture of the drainage. The disease responds to streptomycin.

Brucellosis is usually seen in animals and can be acquired by farmers and animal handlers. Occasionally it is transmitted by unpasteurized milk. The disease is usually mild and self-limited, but it can be treated with trimethoprim–sulfamethoxazole, rifampin, streptomycin, and, except in young children, tetracycline.

TABLE 11–4 · **LESS COMMON CAUSES OF LYMPHADENITIS**

Actinomycosis
Histoplasmosis
Cytomegalovirus
Brucellosis
Bubonic plague
Kawasaki disease
Tularemia
Toxoplasmosis
Sarcoidosis

Acute lymphadenopathy in children younger than 5 years may be the initial presentation of Kawasaki disease (mucocutaneous node syndrome), which is an idiopathic multisystem vasculitis with the potential for developing coronary artery aneurysm and myocardial infarction. Although the disease is rare, it is important to keep it in mind when evaluating children with lymphadenitis, because prompt diagnosis and treatment with aspirin and immunoglobulin can significantly reduce morbidity. Diagnosis requires 5 or more days of fever and four or more of the following accompanying signs: enlarged cervical lymph nodes, conjunctivitis, oral mucosa lesions, polymorphous rash, and characteristic changes of the hands and feet, including pitting edema, periungual desquamation, and erythema of palms and soles.

Other causes of enlarged cervical lymph nodes include sarcoidosis and treatment with certain drugs, such as allopurinol, phenytoin, and hydralazine.

KEY POINTS

— Optimal treatment requires identification of the pathogen.

— Fine-needle aspiration is the most valuable diagnostic test.

— Tuberculous nodes should be treated medically, not excised.

— Nontuberculous mycobacterial nodes should be surgically excised.

— Cat-scratch adenopathy usually resolves without specific therapy.

— Excisional biopsy should be performed if a thorough evaluation fails to demonstrate the cause.

Suggested Readings

White MP, Bangash H, Goel KM, Jenkins PA. Non-tuberculous mycobacterial lymphadenitis. *Arch Dis Child* 61:368–371, 1986.

Zangwill KM, Hamilton DH, Perkins BA, et al. Cat-scratch disease in Connecticut: Epidemiology, risk factors, and evaluation of a new diagnostic test. *N Engl J Med* 329:8–13, 1993.

Congenital Lesions

Congenital neck masses are most often cystic lesions, including thyroglossal duct cyst, branchial cleft cyst, and dermoid cyst. Hemangioma and cystic hygroma are vasuclar malformations that present as soft ballottable neck masses. In a newborn, congenital torticollis presents as a firm neck mass. The diagnosis of a congenital neck mass is usually apparent from the location and consistency of the mass; however, definitive diagnosis of a cyst requires histologic examination of the excised lesion. Surgery plays a smaller role in the management of vascular malformations. Incisional biopsy is contraindicated by the risk of bleeding, and diagnosis is best established by imaging.

Thyroglossal Duct Cyst

In embryologic development, thyroid tissue originates in the base of tongue and then moves downward into the neck, reaching its position by the eighth week. The thyroglossal duct forms during this descent, connecting the thyroid gland to the foramen cecum in the base of the tongue. This duct is normally obliterated during further development, but occasionally a fragment of the duct will persist and form a cyst.

Presentation. A thyroglossal duct cyst most commonly presents as an acutely infected neck mass in the anterior midline of the neck. The average age of presentation in children is 5 years, but approximately 50% of thyroglossal cysts do not present until young adulthood. Sometimes, the mass is detected prior to infection. In other cases, the patient has prior infections that resolved, leaving a persisting cystic mass.

Diagnosis. A thyroglossal duct cyst can usually be recognized on the basis of the physical examination. The characteristic location of this cyst is in the anterior midline of the neck, at or just below the level of the hyoid bone. Occasionally, a thyroglossal cyst will be just to one side of the midline. The cyst moves upward in the neck when the tongue is protruded, because of fibrous duct remnants connecting the cyst to the foramen cecum in the base of the tongue (Fig. 11–3).

Some authors recommend the use of ultrasound or thyroid scanning to detect whether the mass represents the patient's only functioning thyroid tissue. However, this would be a very rare occurrence and could be diagnosed and dealt with at the time of surgical exploration.

Natural History. A thyroglossal duct cyst frequently will undergo cyclical enlargement and shrinkage. In some cases, the mass continues to enlarge, occasionally becoming so quite large that it compresses surrounding structures. The most common clinical problem is infection.

Treatment. A thyroglossal duct cyst should be surgically excised. Because the thyroglossal duct is intimately associated with the hyoid bone, excision of the cyst should include excision of the central portion of the hyoid bone. This practice has been shown to diminish the chance for recurrences of the cyst.

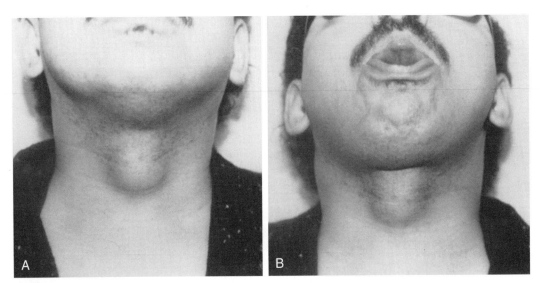

FIGURE 11-3
Anterior view of thyroglossal duct cyst: **A,** patient at rest; **B,** patient protruding the tongue.

Simple surgical excision is generally curative. However, incomplete excision of all thyroglossal duct remnants can result in recurrence. As mentioned above, excision of a recurrent thyroglossal duct cyst is technically difficult, owing to scar tissue and the probable existence of multiple rests of thyroglossal duct tissue. Often, recurrences present with draining fistulas.

Because the best chance for complete excision is during the primary procedure, excision should be performed when the surgical field is in optimal condition—that is, *not* during an acute infection. When a patient presents with an infected thyroglossal cyst, the patient should be treated with antibiotics, with excision planned for 6 or more weeks later. Incision and drainage can create scarring that complicates later definitive surgery; therefore, the cyst should preferably be managed without incision. If necessary, FNA can be performed to decompress an infected cyst and aid in treating the infection.

KEY POINTS

— A thyroglossal duct cyst is a cystic mass in the anterior midline of the neck.

— Most such cysts present in childhood.

— The mass should move upward when the tongue is protruded.

— Treatment is surgical excision.

Suggested Reading

Josephson GD, Spencer WR, Josephson JS. Thyroglossal duct cyst: the New York Eye and Ear Infirmary Experience and a literature review. *Ear Nose Throat J* 77:642–644, 651, 1998.

Branchial Cleft Cysts

Branchial cysts arise from remnants of the embryologic branchial apparatus, which is present during early fetal life. Although frequently regarded to be primordial gills, the branchial arch system actually consists of five mesodermal arches, separated by external clefts and internal pouches. Each arch, with its associated cleft and pouch, comprises a branchial segment, and each segment contributes to the development of specific structures in the head, neck, and upper mediastinum.

The vast majority of branchial cleft lesions arise from the second branchial segment. Second-arch branchial cysts are usually located deep to the anterior border of the sternocleidomastoid muscle, at the level of the hyoid bone. A second-arch sinus will open through the skin along the anterior border of the sternocleidomastoid muscle or into the mouth, just below the tonsil.

Cysts arising from the first branchial segment are relatively uncommon, accounting for approximately 8% of branchial anomalies. They occur in the preauricular region, often in close association to the facial nerve. Fistulas associated with the first cleft open into the external ear canal, or just anterior to it. Third- and fourth-arch lesions arise lower in the neck and are quite rare.

Presentation. Branchial cleft cysts are nearly as common as thyroglossal duct cysts. A branchial cleft cyst typically presents in late childhood or young adulthood, as a lateral neck swelling. Most often the lesion becomes manifest because of an infection. Branchial cleft cysts are sometimes associated with fistulous tracts, which may open either through the skin or mucosa of the mouth or pharynx. When the fistula opens externally, the patient may occasionally note the discharge of milky fluid. Patients with internal fistulas frequently note an occasional foul taste in the mouth.

Diagnosis. Branchial cleft lesions are suspected when a cystic lesion is noted in the lateral neck or preauricular area of a child or young adult. The diagnosis is more certain when there is an associated tract, and therefore the physical examination should include a careful inspection of the skin of the neck, the ear canal, and the preauricular region, as well as the tonsillar fossa.

Imaging is not required for diagnosis. However, if a fistula is present, a radiographic contrast study of the fistula tract is extremely helpful in planning surgery. Computed tomography may be useful in determining the extent of the lesion prior to surgery.

Natural History. Branchial cysts often present when they enlarge during an acute infection (Fig. 11–4). Cysts do not completely regress after resolution of infection, and recurrences of infection are the rule. Draining fistulas may occur.

Treatment. As with other congenital cysts, surgical excision is required. Surgery may be tedious, owing to the need to avoid embryologically related nerves. If a branchial cyst is incompletely excised, there may be troublesome recurrences that are very difficult to manage. Therefore, surgery should be performed under optimal conditions. Excision should not be performed during an infection, and incision and drainage should be avoided. Fine-needle aspiration is very helpful to decompress an acutely infected cyst and hasten resolution.

When to Refer. All branchial cleft cysts should be excised and thus require referral to a surgeon.

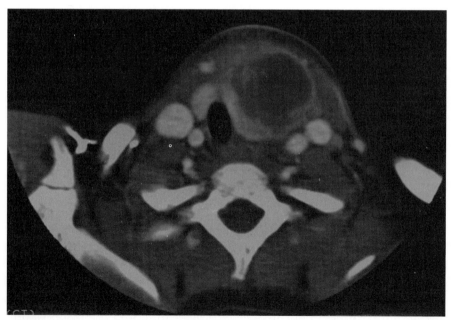

FIGURE 11–4
Computed tomography scan of an infected branchial cleft cyst in a 6-year-old.

KEY POINTS

— Branchial cleft cysts may be associated with fistulous tracts.

— Surgical excision is indicated.

— Cysts often present during an acute infection.

— Surgical excision contraindicated during an acute infection.

— Fine-needle aspiration may be used to drain an acutely infected cyst.

Suggested Reading

Todd NW. Common congenital anomalies of the neck: embryology and surgical anatomy. *Surg Clin North Am* 73:599–610, 1993.

Other Congenital Cysts

Dermoid cysts in the neck generally occur in the midline and therefore may be confused with thyroglossal duct cysts. Like thyroglossal duct cysts, dermoid cysts may present as a painless midline mass or as an acute infection. The chief clinical characteristic that distinguishes these two lesions is that dermoid cysts do *not* move up and down with protrusion of the tongue. Dermoid cysts are composed of both mesodermal and ectodermal tissues and tend to occur along the midline cleft. They differ from "sebaceous" or epidermal inclusion cysts, in that dermoid cysts are located deep to the cervical fascia and therefore are freely movable—not fixed to the skin.

Teratomas are irregular cystic lesions that arise from all three germ layers, each of which may be at differing levels of development. Only 5% of teratomas occur in the head and neck region. Cervical teratomas are usually larger than other congenital masses of the neck and may compress the airway. Teratomas may also arise in the nasopharynx.

Large congenital teratomas can be detected on fetal ultrasound. If airway obstruction is anticipated, a surgeon should be present at delivery to perform urgent tracheotomy if necessary. Ideally, such an infant should be delivered by cesarean section, with preservation of maternal–fetal circulation until an airway is established.

Teratomas should be treated by surgical excision as soon as possible, because of the potential for malignancy. Although teratomas in children are nearly always benign, most of those detected in adults are malignant.

Cystic Hygroma

Cystic hygroma presents as a large, soft, compressible mass, usually in the neck. It is a malformation of lymphatic channels, not connected to the venous system. Because the channels cannot drain, fluid accumulates and dilates the spaces, resulting in apparent growth of the lesion. The lesions are clinically significant when they constitute a visible deformity or when they obstruct the airway.

Approximately 65% of cystic hygromas are apparent at birth, with 90% being detected by the age of 2 years. Often the lesion is first noted when it is enlarged during an URI.

Diagnosis. The diagnosis is frequently established on the basis of findings on physical examination. Cystic hygroma is a diffuse, irregular, soft, compressible, and painless mass, most often in the neck of an infant or small child. Transillumination is pathognomonic, as this is the only lesion in the neck that transilluminates. Magnetic resonance imaging confirms the diagnosis and demonstrates the extent of the lesion. Biopsy is not recommended, as it can result in a chronically draining fistula.

Natural History. These masses are asymptomatic unless there is infection or spontaneous hemorrhage, or unless they compress the airway.

Treatment. Surgical excision, the only effective means of treating this lesion, is usually delayed until after the age of 2. If the lesion compromises the upper airway, a tracheotomy may be indicated, to manage the airway until the child has grown large enough for excision to be feasible. However, if the airway is compromised by tracheal compression, owing to mediastinal involvement, earlier excision may be required.

Surgery should be approached with caution, however, because the lesion tends to be infiltrative, usually extending beyond its clinically apparent borders. It may surround nerves and vascular structures, putting them at risk for injury during surgical excision (Fig. 11–5).

Suggested Reading

Filston HC. Hemangiomas, cystic hygromas, and teratomas of the neck. *Semin Pediatr Surg* 3:147–159, 1994.

Hemangioma

Hemangioma, a proliferative vascular lesion, may present anywhere in the head and neck, including the airway. Approximately 30% of hemangiomas are present at birth, and most of the rest present during

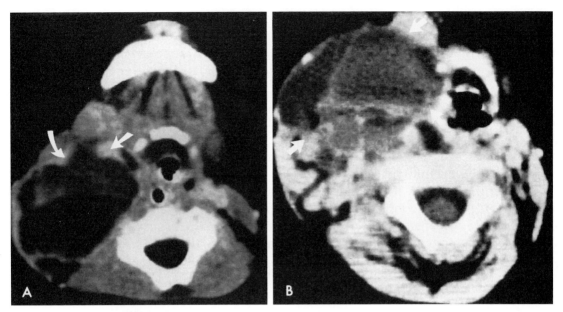

FIGURE 11-5
Computed tomography scans of a cystic hygroma: **A,** in posterior triangle of the neck, with anterior displacement of the carotid sheath structures (*arrows*); **B,** in anterior and posterior triangles of the neck. (From Reede DL, Whelan MA, Bleauox RT. CT of the soft tissue structures of the neck. *Radio Clin North Am* 22:239–250, 1984.)

the first year of life. Often there are multiple lesions. In its most severe form, a large congenital head and neck hemangioma can be a very high flow lesion, resulting in congestive heart failure and consumptive coagulopathy.

Presentation. A hemangioma is a soft, poorly circumscribed mass. When the lesion involves the skin, there is an erythematous or bluish hue. Often there are separate, small cutaneous hemangiomas (strawberry birthmarks). Airway obstruction may develop if the hemangioma extends into the trachea or compresses it.

Diagnosis. Incisional biopsy is contraindicated because of the vascularity of the lesion, and FNA yields only blood cells. Diagnosis is usually established by CT with contrast. Computed tomography is also useful for detecting involvement of the airway.

Natural History. Head and neck hemangioma may be present at birth or appear within the first 2 years of life. Lesions undergo a proliferative phase with a significant increase in size and then begin to regress. The lesions resolve before the age of 7 in about 90% of patients.

Treatment. Unlike cystic hygroma, hemangioma is very likely to resolve spontaneously within a few years. Therefore, a conservative approach is usually warranted, observing for spontaneous regression and reserving treatment for persisting lesions. However, if the hemangioma obstructs the airway or constitutes a significant cosmetic deformity, intervention may be required earlier. Treatment approaches include systemic steroids, intralesional steroids, laser ablation, interferon, and surgical excision.

Surgical excision of head and neck hemangioma is challenging because of the vascularity and infiltrative nature of the lesion. Surgical excision can result in a significant cosmetic or functional deformity, particularly if a large volume of tissue must be resected. Further, hemangioma is an infiltrative lesion, which may involve important structures, such as the facial nerve or the larynx. In such cases, complete surgical resection cannot be accomplished and the involved structures are at considerable risk for injury during the resection. When the hemangioma extends into the lumen of the airway, endoscopic laser ablation is often an effective approach to management. However, intraoperative bleeding can be difficult to control. The wound may heal with scar contracture, resulting in severe airway compromise that is very difficult to correct. For all of these reasons, it is preferable to avoid surgery if possible.

Systemic steroids are sometimes effective in reducing the size of the lesion and hastening spontaneous regression. This approach is particularly helpful in patients with airway compromise. Interferon has also been reported to be effective.

KEY POINTS

— Hemangiomas are soft, compressible masses.

— Most present at birth or during infancy.

— Lesions initially proliferate and then most spontaneously involute.

— Steroids frequently cause regression.

— Surgery is contraindicated unless there is airway obstruction or failure to involute.

Suggested Reading

Hoehn JG, Farrow GM, Devine KD, et al. Invasive hemangiomas of the head and neck. *Am J Surg* 120:495–500, 1970.

Congenital Muscular Torticollis

Congenital torticollis (Fibromatosis colli) is a firm, fibrous neck mass that occurs in newborns. The cause is believed to be intrauterine compression of the venous outflow of the muscle.

Presentation. The deformity may be present at birth or may become evident later. It first appears as a palpable thickening of the muscle and progresses to its maximum size within a month. The mass then regresses, but muscle contracture persists, causing tilting of the head toward the involved side and rotating of the head toward the normal side.

Diagnosis. The diagnosis of congenital torticollis is generally established on the basis of the characteristic physical findings. Sometimes imaging is helpful in confirming the diagnosis. Computed tomography, MRI, and ultrasound can all demonstrate the lesion well. Ultrasound is generally preferred because it is less expensive and does not require patient restraint or sedation. Rarely, FNA cytology may be required to rule out a neoplasm.

Natural History. Without treatment, congenital torticollis interferes with facial and cranial development, leading to mild ipsilateral microsomia.

Treatment. Physical therapy is the initial treatment of choice. The muscle should be passively stretched several times per day. If the mass persists, surgery is indicated. The muscle should be divided or partially excised. After surgery, the neck should be splinted to prevent recurrence of contracture.

When to Refer. If the diagnosis is not clear, surgical consultation is indicated, for consideration of FNA or even open biopsy. Surgical consultation is also in order for torticollis that does not respond to physical therapy.

KEY POINTS

— Congenital torticollis is a fibrous mass in the lateral neck of newborns.

— Palpation can demonstrate the location in the sternocleidomastoid muscle.

— Progressive contracture leads to tilting and rotation of the head.

— The primary treatment is physical therapy.

— Surgery is indicated if physical therapy fails.

Suggested Readings

Lidge RT, Bechol RC, Lambert DN. Congenital muscular torticollis. Etiology and pathology. *J Bone Joint Surg* 39A:1165, 1957.

Tom LWC, Rossiter JL, Sutton LOM, et al. Torticollis in children. *Otolaryngol Head Neck Surg* 105:1–5, 1991.

Tumors

Tumors in the neck are uncommon in children and young adults. However, in a patient older than 40 years, a neck mass is very likely to be a malignant tumor. Benign tumors are much less common and may arise from a variety of cell types. The three most commonly encountered tumor masses in the neck include thyroid tumors, metastatic cancer, and lymphoma.

Thyroid

When a patient presents with a mass in the thyroid gland, the chief clinical concern is the possibility of cancer. The only way to definitively determine whether a nodule is malignant is open biopsy: a partial thyroidectomy. Thyroid nodules are extremely common and can be palpated in between 4% and 20% of asymptomatic patients. Occult thyroid carcinoma is also common and has been found in 10% of autopsy specimens. However, clinically significant thyroid cancer is uncommon, accounting for about 1% of all new cancers diagnosed in the United States each year. Thus, the vast majority of thyroid nodules are benign and do not warrant surgery. One cannot justify the risks and expense of excising every nodule. The clinical objective is to identify those nodules with the greatest risk of cancer. This task has been dramatically altered by the availability of FNA biopsy.

There are different histologic types of thyroid cancer, with varying clinical features to be considered in planning therapy. In general, the prognosis is best for the most common types of tumors. Papillary carcinoma is the most common type of thyroid cancer, accounting for about 80% of all thyroid cancers in the United States. It has a low incidence of systemic metastasis but does tend to spread to cervical lymph nodes. Follicular carcinoma is the second most common type, accounting for approximately 10% of thyroid tumors. Medullary carcinoma of the thyroid is less common. It is associated with hyperplasia of C cells (calcitonin secreting) and is familial in 20% of cases. Finally, anaplastic carcinoma is the least common and most aggressive type of thyroid tumor.

Presentation. Most thyroid nodules are asymptomatic and are detected incidentally during routine examinations by primary physicians. A patient with an autonomously functioning nodule may present with symptoms of hyperthyroidism. More commonly, however, thyroid tumors are nonfunctioning, and tumor-related symptoms are generally the result of compression by the mass. Some patients note only an ill-defined symptom of "something in the neck" or a foreign body sensation in the throat, particularly when swallowing. A large mass may produce symptoms of hoarseness or airway obstruction, owing to compression of surrounding structures.

Diagnosis. In an otherwise asymptomatic patient with a thyroid nodule, the most pressing clinical task is to determine the relative risk of cancer. Information obtained from the medical history and physical examination is helpful in this task. A thyroid nodule in a man or a child of either sex is more likely to be malignant than is a nodule in a woman. Although thyroid cancer is more common in women than in men or children, women are also more likely to have benign thyroid nodules. In both sexes, the incidence of thyroid cancer increases with age. Thus, the risk of malignancy in a given nodule is lowest if the patient is a young woman.

Symptoms of hypo- or hyperthyroidism suggest that a nodule is benign but do not necessarily rule out the possibility of cancer. Hoarseness suggests possible laryngeal paralysis. Although a large benign tumor can compress the recurrent laryngeal nerve, paralysis is more likely to result from invasion of the recurrent laryngeal nerve by malignancy.

A strong risk factor for thyroid cancer is a history of prior radiotherapy. In the 1950s, low-dose irradiation therapy was used for treatment of some benign conditions, such as thymic enlargement and adenoid hypertrophy. The incidence of thyroid cancer in these patients is so high that a thyroid nodule is very likely to be malignant.

Physical characteristics of the mass are also significant. Malignant nodules are usually large, firm, and solitary. Cystic lesions and multiple nodules are much less likely to be malignant.

For many years, radionuclide scanning was the most important diagnostic test used in the evaluation of a thyroid nodule. The most commonly used isotopes are iodine 123 and technetium 99m. A thyroid scan differentiates between "hot" (hyperfunctioning) nodules that take up more isotope and "cold" (hypofunctioning) nodules. The risk of thyroid cancer is greater in a solitary cold nodule than in a functioning hot or warm nodule. However, cancer can and does occur in hot nodules; therefore, scanning is not a definitive test. The value of scanning has diminished markedly in recent years, owing to the availability of FNA, which is much more accurate.

Currently, FNA is the most informative diagnostic test in the evaluation of a thyroid mass. Its sensitivity and specificity are both >90%. It is also inexpensive to perform and involves very little patient discomfort. Fine-needle aspiration produces a better specimen than does large-needle biopsy, with less risk of complications, such as bleeding and tumor seeding. The accuracy is greatly influenced by the experience of both the physician performing the FNA and the cytopathologist interpreting the specimen.

Natural History. Papillary carcinoma is the most common type of thyroid cancer and the most benign. Microscopic papillary cancer is clinically insignificant, as such foci have been found in 10% of autopsied thyroid glands. For papillary carcinoma diagnosed in a clinically palpable nodule, the 30-year cancer death rate is about 6%, despite a recurrence rate of 31%. Cervical metastasis is common, but distant metastasis is rare. Follicular carcinoma of the thyroid has a 30-year cancer death rate of 15%, slightly higher than that for papillary carcinoma. This tumor type is more prone to distant metastasis but less likely to involve the cervical lymph nodes.

Medullary carcinoma of the thyroid tends to metastasize early in its course, to nodes in the neck and mediastinum. Survival rates vary from 60% to 80%.

Anaplastic thyroid cancer has a particularly poor prognosis. It is a rapidly growing and locally aggressive tumor. Complete excision is sometimes impossible because of local invasion. Most series indicate a grim prognosis, but studies reporting the best survival rates indicate that in patients with the cancer, about half of the tumors can be successfully managed by aggressive surgery with postoperative external beam radiation.

Local invasion is the mechanism of death from thyroid cancer. The tumor may obstruct the airway by invading the trachea or may disrupt the spinal cord.

Treatment. If a nodule is asymptomatic and FNA suggests it is benign, no specific treatment has been proven to be necessary, although the administration of thyroid hormone is a generally accepted practice. It is widely believed that the goal of such therapy is to "suppress" the nodule, by reducing the production of endogenous thyroid-stimulating hormone TSH. However, clinical studies indicate that although thyroid suppression reduces the size of functioning thyroid tissue, it has no effect on the size of a cold nodule. Theoretically, the true benefit of thyroid medication is to reduce the chance of future malignancy in the nodule or surrounding gland, by preventing the trophic influence of TSH. L-thyroxin is given, beginning at a dose of 1.6 µg/kg, and increasing to a level sufficient to suppress TSH. Thyroid suppression therapy does carry some risk. The levels of thyroxin necessary to suppress TSH could result in subclinical thyrotoxicosis, which has been associated with the long-term side effects of osteoporosis and cardiomyopathy. Given the potential complications and the lack of documented significant benefits, one can question the indications for thyroid suppression. Whether or not thyroid hormone is given, a thyroid nodule should be monitored carefully and rebiopsied at intervals, particularly if it enlarges.

Surgery may is indicated for the treatment of some nonfunctioning benign thyroid masses or goiter. A very large thyroid mass or goiter can be a significant cosmetic problem. A large mass may also compress the trachea, esophagus, or recurrent laryngeal nerve, resulting in dyspnea, dysphagia, or hoarseness.

When FNA indicates malignancy, then surgery is indicated, to excise the lobe containing the nodule. If histologic examination findings confirm cancer, then usually the opposite lobe should also be removed, with care taken cares to preserve the parathyroid glands. Recurrence of thyroid cancer is significantly higher when a portion of clinically uninvolved gland is left in situ. There are other compelling reasons to remove as much of the gland as possible, depending on the histologic type. Papillary thyroid cancer is frequently multicentric; therefore, if this tumor is found in one lobe, there is a significant risk that there will also be foci of tumor in the opposite lobe. Follicular cancer, the other major subtype of thyroid cancer, behaves differently. Although it is generally not multicentric, it does tend to metastasize, to the bones and to the lungs. These metastases are best managed by systemic administration of radioactive iodine (iodine 131). Such treatment is most efficiently delivered when there is no residual thyroid tissue to take up the iodine. For these reasons, a complete thyroidectomy, followed by thyroid hormone replacement, is recommended.

Complications of thyroid surgery include laryngeal paralysis and, for total or subtotal thyroidectomy, hypoparathyroidism. With currently accepted surgical technique, the incidence of permanent laryngeal paralysis should be <1%, excluding those cases in which the nerve must be sacrificed to completely excise the tumor. The incidence of hypothyroidism is related to the experience of the surgeon in locating and preserving the parathyroid glands during surgery. Permanent hypoparathyroidism is a significant complication, because it requires long-term monitoring of calcium levels and calcium supplementation.

Postoperative iodine 131 is recommended in all but the smallest and best-localized tumors to ablate any healthy thyroid remnant and to reduce the incidence of subsequent pulmonary metastases. Radioactive iodine is not very effective in treating gross residual disease; therefore, surgical resection should be as complete as possible. After ablation with iodine 131, it is possible to use serum thryoglobulin levels and iodine 131 scanning to monitor for recurrence.

Iodine 131 administration requires preparation. To maximize iodine uptake in residual tumor and thyroid tissue, the patient should follow a low-iodine diet for 2 weeks before the scan and the serum TSH should be allowed to rise above 30 μU/ml. To accomplish this, lower doses of thyroid hormone are administered for 1 month after surgery, and then thyroid medication is withheld for the 2 weeks before the test. The patient must be hospitalized until there has been sufficient excretion of the isotope from the system. Treatments should be repeated at 6- to 12-month intervals until no significant uptake is detected or until a large cumulative dose has been reached or until adverse side effects occur. Side effects of iodine 131 include tumor hemorrhage, neck edema, sialadenits, delayed bone marrow damage, and induction of tumors.

Medullary cancer and anaplastic cancer do not respond to iodine 131. Thus, if adjuvant therapy is indicated, the only available option is external beam irradiation.

When to Refer. Patients with benign multinodular goiter require no specific therapy. However, patients with solitary nodules and those with symptoms should be referred for evaluation by a specialist. Optimal management involves collaboration between an endocrinologist and a surgeon (otolaryngologist or general surgeon).

KEY POINTS

— Thyroid nodules are very common.

— Thyroid cancer is uncommon.

— Fine-needle aspiration is the best means of detecting thyroid cancer.

— Prognosis of thyroid cancer is related to histologic type.

— Usual treatment is total thyroidectomy and radioactive iodine.

— A benign thyroid mass should be removed if it impairs breathing or swallowing or is a cosmetic problem.

Suggested Readings

Ezzat S, et al. Thyroid incidentalomas: prevalence by palpation and ultrasonography. *Arch Intern Med* 154:1838–1840, 1994.

Gharib H, et al. Suppressive therapy with levothyroxine for solitary thyroid nodules: A double-blind controlled clinical study. *N Engl J Med* 317:70–75, 1987.

Mazzaferri EL. Management of a solitary thyroid nodule. *N Engl J Med* 328:553–559, 1993.

Yamamoto Y, et al. Occult papillary carcinoma of the thyroid: a study of 408 autopsy cases. *Cancer* 65:1173–1179, 1990.

Metastasis

A painless neck mass in an adult represents malignancy in 85% of cases. Seventy percent of malignant neck nodes are metastatic from tumors of the head and neck, and most of these are squamous carcinoma. Squamous carcinoma occurs is predominantly a disease of older adults, although it does occur in young adults. The vast majority of patients with squamous carcinoma of the head and neck have a significant history of smoking and drinking. Thyroid or salivary gland cancer can also metastasize to lymph nodes in the neck. Rarely, other tumors are involved, such as sarcoma or melanoma. A lymph node in the supraclavicular may contain metastasis from a tumor below the clavicles, such as the lung, breast, kidney, prostate, gonads, or gastrointestinal tract.

Diagnosis. When malignancy is suspected in a cervical lymph node, an important clinical task is to search for a primary tumor in the regions drained by the node so that it can also be treated. A neck mass in a patient with a history of smoking is most likely to be a metastasis from a squamous carcinoma in the mouth or throat. Squamous carcinoma does occur in patients who have not used tobacco or alcohol, but not often, and therefore other primary tumors should be considered.

Clinical symptoms are often useful in locating the site of the lesion. Unilateral hearing loss can result from eustachian tube obstruction by a nasopharyngeal tumor. Ear pain may be referred from a lesion in the pharynx or larynx. Hoarseness, dyspnea, or stridor suggest a laryngeal tumor. A lesion of the pharynx or upper esophagus can cause painful or difficult swallowing. A patient with a lesion in the oral cavity may present with ill-fitting dentures. Hemoptysis is rarely a symptom of a head and neck tumor.

Physical examination of the head and neck examination should include otoscopy. Serous otitis indicates eustachian tube obstruction, which could be caused by a tumor in the nasopharynx. The examination must also inspect all accessible mucosal surfaces in the upper aerodigestive tract. The floor of mouth and base of tongue should also be palpated. Mucosal tumors may present as indurated, ulcerated, or fungating areas. Traditionally, a mirror offers the best view of the nasopharynx and hypopharynx; however, with flexible fiberoptic endoscopy, these areas can be visualized fairly well in most patients. Examination of the neck should note the size and location of the mass and search for the presence of other nodes. The neck mass should be carefully palpated to detect potential fixation to skin or underlying structures. The thyroid and salivary glands should also be carefully examined for nodules.

If a primary site is not noted on physical examination, then FNA biopsy of the mass is indicated. Fine-needle aspiration is 93% sensitive and 97% specific for squamous cell carcinoma. It can also accurately detect many other types of head and neck tumors, including thyroid and salivary gland tumors and lymphoma. If results of FNA are positive for squamous carcinoma or fail to indicate the nature of the neck mass, then the patient must undergo surgical direct endoscopy and directed biopsies to locate the tumor. An otolaryngologist or head and neck surgeon should perform this procedure. Excisional biopsy should not be performed until a thorough search has failed to locate a primary tumor, as optimal management includes treatment of both the primary tumor and the metastases. The node should be excised by a surgeon who is prepared to proceed with further surgery if a tumor is found on intraoperative histologic evaluation of a frozen section.

Natural History. The prognosis for patients with metastatic cancer to the neck is highly variable and is related to the clinical behavior of the primary tumor. Survival is much better for patients with smaller lesions. Thus, early detection is the most important means of improving the survival in these patients.

Treatment. Treatment of metastatic cancer to the neck depends on many factors, including the size of the neck mass, extracapsular spread, the presence of other neck nodes, and the location and stage of the primary tumor. Treatment involves surgery and/or radiation, sometimes in combination with chemotherapy.

If a primary tumor cannot be found as a source of metastatic squamous carcinoma, the accepted treatment is surgical removal of the lymph nodes in the neck (neck dissection). After surgery, radiation therapy is given to the neck and to the areas most likely to contain an occult malignancy responsible for the metastasis. These areas include the nasopharynx, the base of tongue, and the tonsils.

When to Refer. Patients with cervical metastases are best managed by a head and neck oncology team, including a head and neck surgeon and radiotherapist and sometimes a medical oncologist. Any patient with a suspicious neck mass should be referred to a head and neck cancer specialist or an otolaryngologist with training in head and neck cancer.

KEY POINTS

— In an adult who smokes and drinks, the most likely cause of an enlarged cervical lymph node is metastasis from a squamous carcinoma in the head and neck.

— Fine-needle aspiration is used to establish histologic diagnosis.

— Diagnostic workup includes a thorough search for a primary tumor.

Suggested Readings

Martin H, Morfit M. Cervical lymph node metastasis as the first symptom of cancer. *Surg Gynecol Obstet* 78:133, 1994.
Robbins KT, et al. The violated neck: cervical node biopsy prior to definitive treatment. *Otolaryngol Head Neck Surg.* 94:605–610, 1986.

Lymphoma

A neck mass may be the presenting sign of lymphoma. Lymphoma in children is most frequently of the non-Hodgkin's type. During adolescence and young adulthood, Hodgkin's lymphoma is more frequent. Both types of lymphoma become increasingly common after the fifth decade of life.

Presentation. Many patients note "B signs" such as fever, night sweats, or weight loss. The adenopathy of Hodgkin's lymphoma may fluctuate as it gradually increases in size, whereas the nodes of non-Hodgkin's lymphoma (NHL) often grow rapidly. The incidence of NHL is increased in immunocompromised patients.

Diagnosis. Lymphoma presents as a firm, rubbery mass in the neck. It does not regress with a therapeutic trial of antibiotics. In adults, such a mass should be evaluated as a possible metastatic tumor. A complete head and neck examination should be performed to search for a primary tumor. In any age group, FNA should be performed for cytologic evaluation. If cytology suggests lymphoma, then an excisional biopsy is indicated, to allow accurate histologic and immunohistologic classification. This is important in planning therapy.

Other diagnostic testing is important to establish the stage of the disease, including CT of the head and neck, chest, and abdomen. Complete blood count should be performed, and bone marrow biopsy may be indicated. In some cases, staging laparotomy is needed.

Natural History. Hodgkin's disease is usually presents as a slowly growing mass in the neck. It then spreads to contiguous lymph nodes, extending into the mediastimum and then into the abdomen, involving the spleen and subdiaphragmatic nodes, and then the liver and bone marrow. Although Hodgkin's disease is usually confined to lymphatic tissue, NHL is predominantly extranodal, not uncommonly involving the CNS. The growth rate of NHL is variable, depending on the histologic grade.

Treatment. The management of lymphoma depends on the histology and stage. Treatment options include radiation and/or chemotherapy. For early Hodgkin's disease, cure rates are as high as 90%. For advanced disease, only 35% are cured. Survival for patients with NHL ranges from 50% to 80%.

When to Refer. The best survival for patients with lymphoma is achieved by treatment in early stages. Thus, it is crucial to refer patients for evaluation and treatment as soon as it is suspected. Although otolaryngologists and surgeons are involved in diagnosis and staging, therapy is managed by a medical oncologist.

Suggested Reading

Simon R, Durrleman S, Hoppe RT, et al. The non-Hodgkin's lymphoma pathological classification project: long-term follow-up of 1152 patients with non-Hodgkin's lymphomas. *Ann Intern Med* 109:939–945, 1988.

Other Neck Tumors

Several types of uncommon tumors, both benign and malignant, can present as neck masses. These tumors are histologically diverse because they arise from diverse cell types. Even benign neck tumors can cause significant morbidity and mortality, owing to the dense concentration of vital structures in this region.

A group of tumors, called paragangliomas, arise from microscopic neural crest cells in the neck. A family history of similar tumors is found in 10% of patients, and between 20% and 30% of patients have multiple lesions. These tumors are compressible and refill on release of pressure. The mass is frequently pulsatile, with an audible bruit. On microscopic examination, these tumors appear similar to pheochromocytomas; however, head and neck paragangliomas rarely secrete catecholamines. They are, however, highly vascular, and therefor contrast-enhanced CT or MRI usually indicates the diagnosis. Four-vessel angiography is routinely performed to confirm the diagnosis, to establish the blood supply, and to detect other paragangliomas. Vagal paragangliomas arise in the carotid sheath and often the initial sign is laryngeal paralysis due to compression of the vagus nerve. Carotid body tumors have a similar presentation, but angiography demonstrates a characteristic widening of the carotid bifurcation. Glomus jugulare tumors often extend intracranially. Paragangliomas of the middle ear are called glomus tympanicum tumors. Radiotherapy can be effective in some cases, but it primarily slows growth rather than ablating the lesion. Surgical excision is the treatment of choice, but it often results in debilitating paralyses of involved cranial nerves. Because of this surgical morbidity, as well as the fact that the tumors are slow growing and nearly always benign, observation may be the best course of action in elderly asymptomatic patients.

Neurofibromas and schwannomas arise from cells in the nerve sheath. Multiple neurofibromas may arise in patients with von Recklinghausen's disease. As the tumors grow, they compress and infiltrate the associated nerves, with resulting functional deficits. Rarely, these lesions can be malignant. The tumors are radioresistant and therefore surgery is the only effective treatment; however, surgical resection usually causes nerve deficits as well. Therefore, just as in patients with paragangliomas, the risks and benefits of surgery must be weighed in each patient.

Lipomas are encapsulated masses of fatty tissue, most often in the subcutaneous layer. It is not clear whether these are true neoplasms. Treatment is surgical excision. The primary indication for surgery is cosmesis; however, it is also important to rule out atypical lipoma, a locally aggressive benign lesion, and liposarcoma.

12

OTOLARYNGOLOGIC EMERGENCIES

I N T R O D U C T I O N

The vast majority of problems in the ears, nose, and throat are not emergencies and can be evaluated and managed in a routine manner. Infections may be life threatening when the airway or the central nervous system is involved. Infections may also require urgent attention when vision, hearing, and/or balance are in jeopardy. Such infectious problems are addressed in prior chapters, according to the anatomic region involved. This chapter focuses on three specific emergency situations: epistaxis, upper airway obstruction, and aerodigestive tract foreign bodies.

Epistaxis

Nosebleeds are extremely common. The prevalence of acute epistaxis is estimated at 10%–15% of the adult population, whereas the prevalence of chronic recurrent epistaxis is 4%. In the United States, nosebleeds are more frequent during the months of September through April, and this has been attributed to drier and colder air during these months. Among adults there are two peaks in the age distribution, one at 15–25 years, and the second at 45–65 years. Among young children, epistaxis is quite common and is often related to chronic sinus infection.

In the majority of patients with nosebleed, no specific cause can be identified. The most common cause is trauma, including the self-inflicted injuries caused by nose picking.

It is commonly believed that hypertension plays a role in epistaxis. However, studies have found no correlation between hypertension and epistaxis in the general population. It would appear that although hypertension does not increase the occurrence of epistaxis, bleeding tends to be more severe in patients with hypertension. The severity of bleeding has been correlated with the degree of vessel wall disease observed in the retina. It is also true that the stress of a nosebleed often increases blood pressure, so that the bleeding is less likely to resolve spontaneously and is more difficult to control.

Epistaxis is a frequent complication of anticoagulation therapy. The use of aspirin and other nonsteroidal anti-inflammatory drugs also increases the risk of nosebleed. Other medical causes include Osler–Weber–Rendu disease (hereditary hemorrhagic telangiectasia), von Willebrand's disease, and, less commonly, other coagulopathies. Tumors of the nose or nasopharynx may present with nosebleed. Head trauma sometimes results in carotid cavernous sinus fistula, with severe and life-threatening hemorrhage.

Presentation

The majority of nosebleeds are controlled at home. When home remedies fail and patients seek medical attention, the acute bleeding has often subsided by the time they reach the emergency department or a physician's office. Other patients present with a mild to moderate steady flow of blood. Patients use a variety of techniques in attempting to control the bleeding. A common but ineffective approach is to stuff tissue paper into the anterior nostril. The tissue paper does not apply pressure to the bleeding site; it merely dams the blood up inside the nose so that it runs back down the throat or out the other nostril. Some patients present with severe bleeding and may even have signs of shock. Life-threatening nasal hemorrhage is rare and is usually associated with trauma, either acutely or as a late complication.

Diagnosis

The initial diagnostic evaluation is often truncated in patients with epistaxis because of urgent need to control bleeding and/or resuscitate the patient. Therefore, the first step is to establish the severity of the bleeding. The blood loss is usually overestimated by patients because it is frightening to them and because the volume seems much greater when distributed among the various cloths and tissues used in attempting to control the bleeding. Therefore, this clinical judgment should be made on the basis of the amount of active bleeding at the time of presentation and the physical signs of cumulative blood loss, such as orthostasis, tachycardia, hypotension, or pallor. If there are signs of hypovolemia, fluid resuscitation should be instituted concurrently with efforts to stop the bleeding.

The next step is to determine the site of bleeding as accurately as possible (i.e., right vs. left, medial vs. lateral wall, anterior vs. posterior, superior vs. inferior). This information significantly affects the approach to control, as it indicates which cavities should be packed and which blood vessels may need to be embolized or ligated (Fig. 12–1). Physical examination of the nose therefore requires adequate illumination (preferably a headlight or head mirror), a nasal speculum, and suction, to remove all clots and trace the bleeding back to its source. Pathology should also be noted, including septal deformity, mucosal abrasion, or tumor. In profuse epistaxis, it may not be possible to localize bleeding or even to examine the nose. Severe epistaxis often presents bilaterally, even if only one side of the nose is bleeding, as blood flows posteriorly around the septum and out the contralateral nostril.

Certain elements of the medical history are very important in the management of epistaxis. Any history of recent or remote trauma should be noted. A blow to the nose is a common cause of acute epistaxis and may result in nasal fracture. If so, it is critical to determine whether there is a hematoma of the nasal septum. A history of severe head trauma and profuse epistaxis suggests the possibility of a fistula connecting the internal carotid and the cavernous sinus, with onset from weeks to months after the injury.

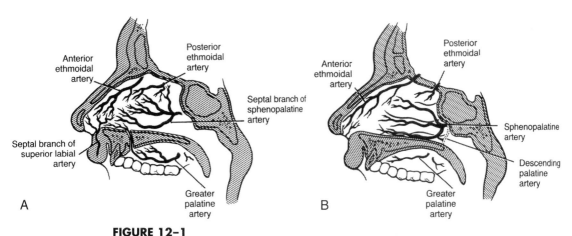

FIGURE 12–1
Blood supply to the nose: **A,** nasal septum; **B,** lateral nasal wall. (From Mabry RL. Nose, paranasal sinuses, and nasopharynx. In Meyerhoff WL, Rice DH [eds]: *Otolaryngology—Head and Neck Surgery,* Philadelphia: WB Saunders, 1992.)

Is this an isolated incident or has the patient had prior bleeding episodes? What has the patient done to try to control the bleeding? The patient should also be questioned about chronic obstructive symptoms that could indicate a septal deformity, chronic sinus infection, or tumor.

The patient should be specifically asked about anticoagulant medication. Epistaxis does occur as a complication of appropriate therapy, but it may also be a sign of anticoagulation. The medical indication for anticoagulation should also be established, so that the risk of discontinuing anticoagulation (for control of acute bleeding) can be assessed.

Treatment

Nosebleeds can nearly always be controlled by a stepwise approach, progressing from simple to more invasive techniques. These steps are detailed in Table 12–1. First, as mentioned in the section on diagnosis, the nose should be carefully inspected to identify the site of bleeding. Usually, this requires suctioning of blood and clots from the nasal cavity. The examination is facilitated by the use of topical anesthesia for patient comfort, and vasoconstriction to decrease blood flow and improve visualization. Cocaine was long preferred as a topical agent because it is the only local anesthetic that also acts as a potent vasoconstrictor. However, owing to toxicity and concerns related to the abuse potential of the drug, topical xylocaine (4%) is preferred, combined with Neo-Synephrine or oxymetazoline for vasoconstriction. In many cases of mild epistaxis, removal of clots and the use of topical vasoconstriction suffice to control the bleeding.

The most common site for nosebleeds is the anterior nasal septum. This area has a rich blood supply and is frequently exposed to trauma. Moderate bleeding in this area may often be controlled with local cautery, using silver nitrate or electrocautery, treating the bleeding vessel and surrounding mucosa to a 2- to 3-mm radius. For either method to be effective, active bleeding should be continuously suctioned away during cautery.

TABLE 12–1 • **STEPS IN MANAGING EPISTAXIS**

1. Removal of blood and clots from nasal cavity
2. Topical vasoconstriction and anesthesia
3. Compression of external nose against septum
4. Local cautery
5. Local packing with absorbable material
6. Anterior nasal packing
7. Posterior packing (always combined with anterior packing)
8. Surgical or angiographic intervention

If cautery is unsuccessful or if bleeding appears to be arising from a more posterior site that is inaccessible to cautery, the next step is packing. For mild to moderate epistaxis, a small piece of absorbable material, such as gelatin foam or cellulose, may be adequate, wedged between septum and turbinate. In other cases, a formal pack is required, filling one or both nasal cavities. Prefabricated nasal packs are currently available in most emergency departments, composed of compressed polymer material. These are relatively easy to use, but it is usually necessary to trim the pack to fit. The depth of the nasal cavity can be measured by passing the suction along the floor of the nose to the back of the septum and then noting the point on the suction opposite the collumella. The distance between this point and the tip of the suction should be the length of the cellulose pack. The pack should be lubricated lightly with antibiotic ointment or cream, to retard bacterial overgrowth and facilitate ultimate removal. However, the pack should not be significantly hydrated prior to placement, as this will result in premature expansion. A bayonet forceps should be used to gently slide the pack into the nose, parallel to the septum. Ongoing bleeding usually saturates the pack so that it expands to fill the nasal cavity. If not, then 1–2 mL sterile saline should be instilled. If a unilateral pack on the side of active bleeding is not sufficient, the next step is to pack the opposite nasal cavity, as this stabilizes the septum and increases the pressure within the bleeding cavity.

Other prefabricated devices are marketed to control epistaxis, such as intranasal balloons. Balloons generally do not conform well to the shape of the nasal cavity. Thus, pressure may not be localized over the bleeding site or may be excessive.

When prefabricated packing is not available or is not sufficient to control the bleeding, an old-fashioned ribbon gauze pack should be used; 0.5-in. gauze should be impregnated with antibiotic ointment or cream and then placed into the nasal cavity in layers. The nostril should be dilated with an nasal speculum and the gauze should be grasped at about 15–20 cm from its end, using bayonet forceps, and advanced all the way through the nasal cavity, leaving some of the free end to exit the nostril (Fig. 12–2). This results in a double layer of gauze in the nose. With the speculum used to stabilize the first layer, a second layer should be added, and the same process should be followed to add successive layers, until the bleeding is controlled or no more gauze can be packed in. As with the prefabricated packs, unilateral packing is often insufficient, and both sides of the nose should usually be packed.

When anterior packing fails, the next step is a posterior pack. This is true even when the bleeding is located anteriorly. A posterior pack fills the nasopharynx to form a posterior support for the anterior pack, increasing the pressure that can be generated in the nasal cavity. *A posterior pack for epistaxis should never be used in isolation but should always be combined with anterior packing.*

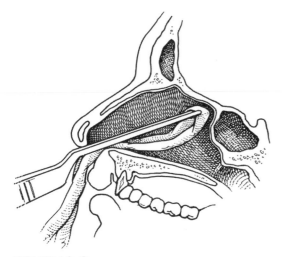

FIGURE 12-2
Technique of nasal packing. (From Mabry RL. Nose, paranasal sinuses, and nasopharynx. In Meyerhoff WL, Rice DH [eds]: *Otolaryngology—Head and Neck Surgery,* Philadelphia: WB Saunders, 1992.)

The most efficient way to place a posterior pack is to pass a Foley catheter with a large (30-mL) balloon through one nostril and into the nasopharynx. The balloon is then inflated with sufficient water to prevent the catheter from being pulled back through the posterior choana. Alternative materials for a posterior pack include lamb's wool or gauze, secured with umbilical tape. Anterior traction is used to wedge the balloon or pack against the posterior choana while bilateral anterior packing is placed.

A posterior pack depresses the soft palate and can partially obstruct the upper airway. Posterior packing has been associated with hypoxia and sudden death; therefore, all patients who require a posterior pack should be admitted to the hospital for monitoring and supplemental oxygen.

Prophylactic antibiotics should be administered. Nasal packing blocks mucus drainage and the resulting collection of blood and inspissated mucus forms a rich culture medium for bacteria. Thus, in the absence of antibiotics, the packing will quickly become foul-smelling and sinusitis is common. Toxic shock syndrome is a rare but potentially fatal complication of nasal packing. Penicillin is usually adequate to coverage, but broad-spectrum antibiotics may be indicated in hospitalized patients or those who have been taking antibiotics recently. Packing should be left in place for at least 3–4 days. Premature removal may result in even more severe epistaxis, as any type of packing results in mucosal injuries that will also bleed. After pack removal, patients should be educated to avoid nasal trauma and keep the nasal cavity moist with saline nose spray or steam inhalation. They should also be instructed in how to use external pressure to control recurrent bleeding.

In addition to control of active bleeding, a major priority in the management of epistaxis is the assessment and treatment of blood loss. Although blood replacement is not often required for patients with epistaxis, severe bleeding can occasionally result in hypovolemic shock, and rarely, death. Moreover, patients who are chronically ill or those with chronic recurrent epistaxis may have anemia, which makes them less tolerant of a modest acute loss of blood. For patients who are already ill or those who have significant bleeding, management requires attention to vital signs, complete blood count and clotting studies, and replacement of fluids or even blood products if indicated. Complete blood count should be repeated after fluid replacement and after there has been enough time for equilibration.

When to Refer

Urgent consultation is indicated when acute bleeding cannot be controlled by cautery or anterior packing. In many cases, an effective anterior pack placed by an experienced otolaryngologist will suffice and the patient will be spared the morbidity of a posterior pack. If the patient does require a posterior pack, hospitalization is required for monitoring.

When packing fails, the options are either surgery or radiographic embolization. Occasionally, the septum is too crooked to permit packing and a septoplasty is required. More often, surgical intervention consists of arterial ligation. Earlier in the twentieth century, external carotid ligation was standard practice, but through the years, the site of intervention has moved closer to the nose. The internal maxillary artery supplies the anterior and inferior portions of the nose, the areas most often involved in bleeding. This vessel can be ligated by an approach through the maxillary sinus. A potential complication of this approach is infraorbital nerve damage. More recently, a technique has been reported for ligating this artery using intranasal endoscopy. This technique requires extensive endoscopic experience and is obviously impossible when bleeding is profuse. For posterior bleeding, the ethmoidal arteries can be ligated.

Embolization is another option. Percutaneous angiography is used to localize feeding arteries and embolize with various materials: coils, Gelfoam, and polyvinyl alcohol. Complications include blindness, stroke, and skin necrosis.

After control of acute epistaxis, referral is often indicated for follow-up care. A single minor episode does not warrant an extensive evaluation, but a patient with severe or recurring epistaxis may have underlying pathology, such as chronic sinusitis, a tumor, an aneurysm, or bleeding diathesis. In children, chronic epistaxis is frequently related to chronic sinusitis or adenoiditis. Antibiotic therapy is indicated and usually quite effective. If recurrent epistaxis persists, surgery, such as septoplasty or septal dermoplasty, may be required.

KEY POINTS

— Epistaxis is extremely common and usually can be controlled at home.

— Epistaxis prompting an emergency-department visit is usually anterior and is easily controlled by local cautery or anterior packing.

— It is important to localize the site of bleeding as accurately as possible and use the least morbid form of treatment.

— If anterior packing fails, the next step is *anterior and posterior* packing, with hospitalization for monitoring.

— Posterior packing should always be used in combination with anterior packing.

— In some patients, bleeding cannot be controlled by cauterization or packing and requires embolization or surgery.

— A single easily controlled episode of epistaxis does not warrant extensive evaluation, but patients with severe or recurrent bleeding should be referred to an otolaryngologist.

— The most common cause of recurrent epistaxis in a child is chronic sinus or adenoid infection.

— Rarely, nasal hemorrhage is life threatening, as in patients with traumatic carotid–cavernous sinus fistula or tumors.

Suggested Readings

Mabry RL. Management of epistaxis by packing. *Otolaryngol Head Neck Surg* 94:401–403, 1986.

Strong EB, Bell DA, Johnson LP, Jacobs JM. Intractable epistaxis: Transantral ligation vs. embolization: Efficacy review and cost analysis. *Otolaryngol Head Heck Surg* 113:674–678, 1995.

Weiss NS. Relation of high blood pressure to headaches, epistaxis, and selected other symptoms. *N Engl J Med* 287:631–633, 1972.

Airway Obstruction

Acute upper airway obstruction is one of the more frightening and challenging emergencies encountered in clinical practice. Quick action is required, because even a few minutes of anoxia can result in brain damage or death. Sound judgment and skill are also critical. If the wrong technique is selected for establishing the airway or if a technical error is made, the consequences may be fatal.

Presentation

Upper airway obstruction is characterized by inspiratory stridor. The onset may be gradual, as in patients with tumor or stenosis. Rapidly progressive stridor is characteristic of acute infectious processes, such as epiglottitis. Trauma can cause sudden severe obstruction, which may be immediate or delayed. Aspirated food may cause sudden total upper airway obstruction (café coronary).

Diagnosis

The urgent need to establish an airway often precludes any real diagnostic activity. However, it is important to assess as efficiently as possible the level and severity of obstruction as well as the cause of the problem, because optimal management is dictated by this information.

Level of Obstruction. Stridor is the key physical finding that distinguishes upper airway obstruction and differentiates patients with obstruction from those with pulmonary dyspnea. Inspiratory stridor indicates obstruction at or above the glottis. With fatigue or severe glottic narrowing, stridor may be biphasic. By contrast, intrathoracic airway obstruction causes noise during expiration. This is because intrathoracic pressure rises during exhalation, resulting in airway collapse.

Severity. Severity is best judged by assessing the degree of effort in breathing in relation to the volume of air exchange. Physical signs of increased inspiratory effort include the use of accessory muscles of respiration (cervical strap muscles, intercostal muscles) and inspiratory suprasternal or intercostal retraction. Restlessness is another important physical sign of the severity of airway obstruction, as patients become confused and agitated with hypoxia.

The noise of stridor is the most obvious physical sign of obstruction, but the loudness of the stridor does not correlate reliably with the severity of obstruction. Many patients with severe obstruction quickly notice that rapid inspiration collapses the airway; therefore, compensatory slowing of inhalation is common. With long, slow inspiration, the volume of air exchanged can be optimized. On the other hand, some patients panic and breathe too rapidly in their struggle to breathe, so that stridor is louder. Finally, if a patient is fatigued, breathing effort may be markedly reduced, so that stridor is mild, even when the airway is nearly completely obstructed. In fact, decreasing stridor may be an ominous sign of decompensation and pending respiratory arrest.

As time permits, a limited medical history and physical examination should be performed to determine the cause of the obstruction and the best means of relieving that obstruction. In an acute trauma victim, airway obstruction suggests a possible fracture of the larynx or even a laryngotracheal separation. Signs of infection, such as fever and chills, suggest possible epiglottitis or perhaps an abcess in the floor of the mouth or deep neck space. Acute burns, from inhalation or caustic ingestion, may also cause airway obstruction. A history of prior intubation raises the possibility of subglottic or tracheal stenosis. Acute stridor may rarely be the presenting sign of a neurologic disorder, such as myasthenia gravis or parkinsonism. Finally, it should be remembered that stridor is sometimes a psychiatric symptom, associated with voluntary adduction of the glottis during inspiration.

The neck should be examined externally for signs of infection, trauma, or tumor. Subcutaneous air indicates communication between the airway and soft tissue, such as a tracheal tear, laryngeal fracture, or rupture of a bronchus or the esophagus. The "Adam's apple" may be distorted or obscured by hematoma if there is a laryngeal fracture. A large neck node or thyroid tumor may displace and compress the trachea.

The safest way to evaluate the lumen of the upper airway is with a flexible nasopharyngoscope, using topical anesthesia. Attempts to use a laryngeal mirror can cause gagging, which may lead to sudden, total airway obstruction. Any obstructing masses or edema should be noted, and the larynx should be assessed for normal opening and closing with respiration.

Other Tests. Blood gas assessment is indicated to establish the degree of respiratory distress and need for intervention. Some radiographs are indicated, but a patient with significant respiratory distress should not be sent to the radiology department unless accompanied by a physician capable of establishing airway patency. A chest x-ray is important, with particular attention to possible causes of sudden airway distress, including pneuothorax, pneumomediastinum, or segmental hyperinflation or collapse. In some cases, a soft-tissue lateral radiograph is helpful in evaluating the subglottis and supraglottis. Computed tomography scanning should be used only when the airway is stable and when findings will influence treatment.

Treatment

Management of airway obstruction ranges from observation to supportive care to airway intervention. If it appears that the problem is likely to be temporary and not life threatening, mere observation may be in order. However, when airway distress is severe enough for the patient to seek medical attention, some form of supportive medical care is usually indicated. Observation and supportive care should take place in an environment where the patient is continuously monitored and personnel and equipment for airway intervention are immediately available. Oxygen, humidification, and steroids are the mainstays of supportive care. Intermittent treatment with nebulized racemic epinephrine may be effective in reducing mucosal edema and improving airway patency.

An oral airway or a nasopharyngeal trumpet can be helpful when the obstruction is due to loss of tone in upper airway muscles. This situation is frequently encountered in patients recovering from a general anesthetic or in any situation that impairs consciousness. A nasopharyngeal airway is a soft trumpet-shaped tube that is passed through one nostril and extends beyond the soft palate into the hypopharynx. An oral airway is a rigid, curved appliance, designed to be between the teeth anteriorly and to extend backward, creating a space between the tongue and the palate and posterior pharyngeal wall.

The Heimlich maneuver should be used in a conscious patient with sudden, total airway obstruction, particularly when this occurs during eating. In such cases, a laryngeal foreign body should be strongly suspected. A Heimlich maneuver uses forceful compression of residual air in the lungs to generate sufficient subglottic pressure to eject the foreign body. It is a standard technique included in basic life support courses and illustrated on placards in most public restaurants. For best results, the rescuer should stand behind the victim and clasp arms around the abdomen, just below the xyphoid or over the sternum, then suddenly squeeze. Pressure can also be applied to a recumbent victim. The Heimlich maneuver should also be used in an unconscious nonbreathing patient who cannot be passively ventilated because of total airway obstruction.

Temporizing Measures. Sometimes airway intervention is clearly indicated but personnel and equipment are not immediately available. Some authors have recommended passing several large-bore needles through the cricothyroid membrane, or at any available location, into the trachea to buy time until a definitive airway can be established. This provides incremental improvement and may be better than doing nothing, but it does not provide adequate ventilation. A more physiologic solution is to have the patient breathe heliox, a mixture of oxygen in helium that can provide rapid and dramatic improvement in ventilation. This gas mixture is much less dense than oxygen in air (or even 100% oxygen) and hence flows much more easily through narrowed passages. Neither of these approaches has any value if there is no spontaneous respiratory activity.

Another temporizing option is the use of transtracheal needle ventilation. This provides rapid access to the airway and may be used until a more definitive airway is established. A 16-gauge needle is passed through the skin and into the trachea, preferably through the cricothyroid membrane. Optimally, an intravenous catheter should be used, so that the rigid needle can be removed, leaving a plastic catheter in place. Placement in the airway is confirmed by aspirating air. The needle is then connected to an oxygen line equipped with an airflow interrupter and providing 50 lb/sq in pressure. By intermittently releasing the interrupter, air can be forced into the trachea. It is important to ensure adequate outflow of air between inflation; otherwise, dangerously high intrapulmonary pressure will be created, compromising venous return and possibly leading to pneumothorax or pneumomediastinum. Inadequate air egress can also result in carbon dioxide retention. Other potential risks of this technique include injection of air outside the trachea, into tissues. This can result in subcutaneous emphysema, pneumothorax, or pneumomediastinum.

Establishing an Airway. Several techniques can be used to establish an airway (Table 12–2). It is crucial to selection of the appropriate technique for securing the airway, and the most experienced person available should perform the intervention. For example, if the obstruction is within the trachea, a cricothyrotomy will enter the airway above the obstruction. An unsuccessful attempt to orotracheally intubate a patient can convert a partial obstruction to total occlusion.

It is very important to preserve spontaneous ventilation whenever possible. In a patient struggling to maintain a marginal airway, paralysis, general anesthesia, or even sedation commonly results in collapse of the airway, owing to inactivaction of the upper airway dilating muscles. Thus, a difficult situation suddenly becomes critical. If controlled ventilation cannot be established quickly, brain damage or death will result. Exceptions may sometimes be made to this rule (e.g., children with suspected epiglottitis) but only when the patient is in the operating suite, with personnel and equipment immediately available for all forms of airway intervention.

TABLE 12–2 • **STEPS IN MANAGEMENT OF AIRWAY OBSTRUCTION**

Sudden, complete
1. Heimlich maneuver
2. Oropharyngeal sweeps
3. Repeated Heimlich maneuver
4. Cricothyrotomy

Partial obstruction, comatose patient
1. Head extension
2. Jaw thrust
3. Pharyngeal airway
4. Airway intervention

Partial obstruction, conscious patient
1. Determination of site, severity, and cause of obstruction
2. Administration of supplemental oxygen
3. Administration of steroids and/or racemic epinephrine
4. Administration of heliox
5. Airway intervention

Orotracheal intubation is the most commonly used technique for establishing an airway (Table 12–3). This approach is impossible when the larynx cannot be exposed, owing to bleeding, secretions, or severe edema in the mouth and/or pharynx. Standard orotracheal intubation requires extension of the neck to expose the larynx and is thus hazardous in patients with potential cervical spine injuries.

Blind nasotracheal intubation should *not* be attempted without experience with the technique and confidence in one's ability to perform it, unless there is no other option. The tube is passed through the nose and then guided into the larynx by listening to airflow from the tube orifice. This is a risky method of establishing an airway, and it is even more difficult and hazardous in the setting of acute upper airway obstruction.

Flexible endoscopy should be used to guide intubation when standard exposure is difficult. The endoscope is passed through the endotracheal tube and then through the mouth or nose and on into the trachea. When the endoscope is well into the trachea, the endotracheal tube is advanced over it. The endoscope is withdrawn after ensuring that the endotracheal tube is incorrect position.

Nasal or orotracheal intubation by any method of exposure is risky when the larynx and/or trachea are injured. The tube may enter a laceration, creating a false passage, or converting a partial tracheal transection to total separation. A cricothyrotomy may also be difficult in the presence of laryngeal or tracheal trauma, as landmarks are obscured, and there may be obstruction distal to the subglottis. Thus, the safest means of establishing an airway in such patients is an emergency tracheotomy. With experience, a tracheotomy can often be performed in 1 or 2 minutes.

A cricothyrotomy should be performed when seconds count, because obstruction is total, or when no one is available who can

---

TABLE 12–3 • **OPTIONS FOR AIRWAY INTERVENTION IN UPPER AIRWAY OBSTRUCTION**

Tracheal intubation
   Orotracheal
   Blind nasal
   Fiberoptically guided

Transtracheal needle
   Spontaneous breathing
   Jet ventilation

Cricothyrotomy

Tracheotomy

Rigid bronchoscopy

perform an emergency tracheotomy. First, the head is extended (unless a cervical spine injury is suspected). The thyroid and cricoid cartilages are identified by palpation. A horizontal stab incision is made through the skin and into the airway in the space between these two cartilages. A number 11 scalpel blade is ideal, but in urgent circumstances, nearly any sharp object will do. After making the incision, the blade is rotated 90° to open the space. Something should be passed into the trachea to secure the airway. This could be a tracheotomy or endotracheal tube, but even the hub of a ballpoint pen can be used.

Cricothyrotomy is a rapid and reliable means of establishing an airway in most patients. However, it is sometimes difficult to identify the laryngeal cartilages. They can be obscured by obesity or by overlying inflammation or tumor. In children, the cartilages are soft and indistinct. Cricothyrotomy should not be performed unless the proper landmarks can be confidently identified, as incising in the wrong location could have a disastrous outcome. If the incision is too high, the larynx will be damaged and the airway will not be secured. If the incision is too lateral, nerves and vessels of the carotid sheath may be damaged. If the incision is too low, it could involve the thyroid gland, with potentially severe bleeding. When the landmarks cannot be identified, then the skin should be incised vertically in the midline and the trachea or cricothyroid membrane should be identified and incised by open dissection.

Sometimes the only viable option for establishment of an airway is rigid bronchoscopy. This is most often encountered in patients with tracheal obstruction, owing to tumor, stenosis, or tracheomalacia. Endotracheal intubation may be impossible in these patients, because the tube cannot be forced through the obstruction. And often, the obstruction is distal to the endotracheal tube, so that the airway is still obstructed. In such cases, a rigid bronchoscope allows dilation of the airway. It can be passed all the way to the carina, or even into a mainstem bronchus, using direct visualization.

When to Refer

In acute upper airway obstruction, the airway should be established by the most experienced person available. Anesthesiologists and critical care specialists are highly skilled in intubation and are trained to handle difficult airways. Otolaryngologists also have expertise in emergency airway management, particularly in performing tracheotomy or rigid bronchoscopy. Unfortunately, airway emergencies frequently arise when no specialist is availble. Thus, all physicians should have basic skills in endotracheal intubation and cricothrotomy.

KEY POINTS

— The characteristic physical sign of upper airway obstruction is stridor.

— The first priority in managing upper airway obstruction is to determine the level and severity of the obstruction.

— If obstruction is sufficiently severe to warrant airway intervention, this should be performed by the most experienced person available.

— Sedation, paralysis, or general anesthesia should be avoided until a stable airway has been established.

— A cricothyroidotomy is the most rapid means of establishing a stable airway.

Suggested Readings

Spait DW, Joseph M. Prehospital cricothyrotomy: an investigation of indications, technique, complications, and patient outcome. *Ann Emerg Med* 13:273–285, 1990.
Watson CB. A survey of intubation practices in critical care medicine. *Ear Nose Throat* 62:494–501, 1983.

Foreign Bodies in the Esophagus and Airway

Airway foreign bodies cause thousands of deaths per year. When an object totally occludes the larynx, no airflow is possible, resulting in death within minutes. If the object is irregularly shaped, it may not completely occlude the larynx but may result in partial obstruction and inspiratory stridor.

If a foreign body is small enough to pass through the glottis, it will not totally obstruct the trachea, but it can cause significant airway distress, with characteristically biphasic stridor. This obstruction is progressive, owing to edema and retained mucus. Bronchial foreign bodies in general do not result in sudden death or significant sustained dyspnea; however, delayed death may result from chronic infection and the body's response to the foreign body. The lung distal to a bronchial foreign body may become hyperinflated, owing to a "ball–valve effect." Air flows in during inspiration, when negative intrathoracic pressure distends the bronchus, but during expiration, intrathoracic pressure rises and the bronchus collapses around the foreign body, resulting in restricted airflow (expiratory wheeze) or total obstruction of that airway segment. With time, local inflammation can convert this one-way valve into total obstruction, with collapse of the lung tissue distal to it.

Esophageal foreign bodies cause less morbidity. Most swallowed objects pass uneventfully through the digestive tract, but passage may be restricted if the object is large or if there is esophageal pathology. There are three common sites of esophageal impaction: the cricopharyngeus and the areas of extrinsic compression by the aorta and left mainstem bronchus. Sharp objects may perforate the esophagus, leading to life-threatening mediastinitis.

Small children have a tendency to place inappropriate things into their mouths, and most foreign bodies are aspirated or swallowed small objects, such as coins, safety pins, or crayons. Airway obstruction may result from ingestion of a food that the child is not developmentally prepared to chew and swallow. Before the age of 3 years, children lack molars and are unable to crush nuts; thus, peanuts are a common bronchial foreign body in young children. The foods most often responsible for laryngeal obstruction and sudden death in children are hot dogs, grapes, and peanut butter. Many tragic deaths could be avoided by education of parents about this danger.

A particularly hazardous foreign body, increasingly a culprit in airway obstruction, is the small disc battery. When lodged in the esophagus, these batteries can cause severe local tissue destruction, owing to the release of concentrated sodium or potassium hydroxide; thus, removal is urgently indicated.

In adults, most foreign bodies are from ingested food, such as fish bones, chicken bones, or poorly chewed meat. Sudden laryngeal obstruction is termed a café coronary. Decreased intraoral sensation, dentures, and inebriation contribute to foreign body ingestion in adults. An esophageal foreign body may also be the presenting sign of an esophageal tumor or reflux esophagitis.

Presentation

Complete sudden airway obstruction may or may not be preceded by coughing or choking. Once the airway is totally occluded, however, speech and coughing are impossible. No air moves in or out, despite strong breathing efforts. Although silent, the victim is usually agitated and in obvious distress, often gesturing at the obstruction by grabbing or pointing to the throat. After several minutes, unconsciousness follows, owing to anoxia. This is an absolute emergency, as death occurs within minutes without intervention.

Inspiratory stridor and hoarseness are the characteristic physical signs of partial laryngeal obstruction. Tracheal foreign bodies are associated with "biphasic" stridor, in both inspiration and expiration. Presence of a foreign body in either location induces edema, which may progress to total obstruction.

The classic triad of signs associated with a bronchial foreign body are coughing, wheezing, and decreased breath sounds. However, not all patients exhibit all or even any of these signs. The actual event of aspiration of the object into the airway is associated with coughing and choking, but these symptoms quickly subside. In most cases, an asymptomatic interval follows, as the object comes to rest in a bronchus. Symptoms of wheezing and coughing begin to appear at variable intervals, owing to local edema, infection, and/or granulation tissue.

Esophageal foreign bodies present with inability to swallow and frequently substernal discomfort or frank pain. Drooling is common. There may be a history of gagging or choking. Quite commonly, the local trauma from a swallowed foreign body will produce pain or obstructive symptoms that persist for hours or even days after the object has passed.

Diagnosis

Sudden upper airway obstruction is easy to identify while the patient is still conscious. As mentioned above, the patient is agitated, restless, and unable to utter a sound. Frequently, gestures are made to communicate the problem, including pointing to the neck and placing the hands around the neck to mimic choking. Once the patient is unconscious and respiratory efforts cease, the problem is no longer apparent. Airway obstruction should always be considered in any case of sudden respiratory arrest. Immediate attempts to restore the airway take precedence over any diagnostic activity.

In patients with partial upper airway obstruction, intervention is not immediately necessary, and some time can be afforded for further evaluation. Sometimes there is a clear history of choking on an object. The level of obstruction can generally be inferred by the timing of the stridor. Inspiratory stridor indicates laryngeal obstruction, whereas expiratory stridor indicates intrathoracic obstruction. Biphasic stridor is characteristic of tracheal obstruction or of severe obstruction at any level. Auscultation of the trachea and chest are very useful in localizing the obstruction.

The nose and mouth should be examined directly. The vallecula and the inferior tonsil are common sites for a fish bone to lodge, and a foreign body at these locations can often be identified by transoral inspection. Fish bones are often transparent and may appear to be a strand of saliva or mucus. Flexible endoscopy, using topical anesthesia, is the safest means of examining the hypopharynx and larynx. With the exception of an occasional subglottic obstruction, foreign bodies beyond the larynx cannot be visualized on physical examination.

Sudden inability to swallow prompts a presumptive diagnosis of an esophageal foreign body. The diagnosis is strengthened when there is drooling or substernal discomfort. The history may indicate the obstructing object, most frequently meat or bones in adults. Children may have been observed to place small objects into the mouth, but most foreign-body ingestion by children is not witnessed.

Dysphagia and local pain, in the absence of actual obstruction, are less compelling signs of the presence of a foreign body. As mentioned above, these symptoms commonly persist for a day or so after a foreign body is swallowed and passed on. However, if symptoms persist longer, the possibility of a retained foreign body is increased.

Radiologic examination should include anteroposterior and lateral views of the neck and chest. Occasionally a radiopaque foreign body can be seen on a soft-tissue x-ray. Objects with very distinctive shapes, such as safety pins, are easily identified. In particular, coins are very easily seen. Small disc batteries are easily recognized, as they appear as double discs. Many foreign bodies are radiolucent, and often, calcifications in ligaments are mistaken for foreign bodies.

The appearance of a coin on chest x-ray indicates its location, in the trachea or esophagus. A coin in the trachea is most likely to lie in an anteroposterior plane. The trachea has cartilage rings that are deficient posteriorly. Thus, the coin lies in an anteroposterior plane because it displaces the soft posterior tracheal wall. On anteroposterior view, a coin in the trachea will be seen on edge; it will be seen as a disc on lateral view. By contrast, a coin in the esophagus will lie in a coronal plane so that it appears as disc on anteroposterior view and is seen on edge on lateral view.

Chest films are very important in evaluating a patient with a suspected bronchial foreign body, but not to visualize the foreign body itself. Either fluoroscopy or static films in both inspiration and expiration are used to demonstrate the effects of the foreign body on ventilation. If there is a ball–valve effect of the foreign body, the affected lung will remain inflated during expiration (Fig. 12–3). In some cases, the resulting air trapping leads to hyperinflation, with mediastinal shift to the opposite side. Bronchial foreign bodies can also completely block a bronchus, so that air absorption leads to atelectasis.

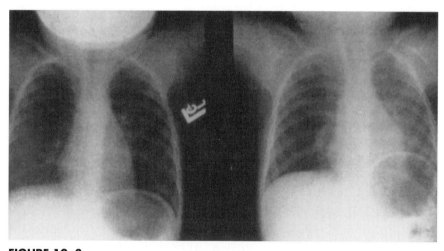

FIGURE 12–3
Chest x-ray in inspiration (*left*) and expiration (*right*), demonstrating air trapping distal to a bronchial foreign body in the right bronchus.

Natural History

Foreign bodies in the lower respiratory tract are rarely coughed out. Most remain lodged, leading to increasing obstruction with local inflammation and infection. In particular, a bronchial foreign body can lead to severe recurring infections with bronchiectasis. Prior to the development of endoscopic retrieval, mortality was high.

By contrast, pharyngeal or esophageal foreign bodies are more benign. The majority of foreign bodies are eventually passed through the gastrointestinal tract. Foreign bodies frequently cause local trauma in the pharynx or esophagus, and the resulting pain or obstructive symptoms can persist for hours or days after the foreign body has passed. On occasion, however, a foreign body may be chronically lodged in the esophagus and may be manifested by such symptoms as weight loss, fever, or vomiting.

Treatment

Foreign bodies that have been swallowed and passed into the stomach and beyond can usually be monitored until they pass from the body spontaneously. Exceptions would include sharp objects with the potential for perforation. Foreign bodies in the airway or those lodged in the esophagus should be removed. The preferred means for removal is via rigid endoscopy, with direct visualization under general anesthesia.

Alternative techniques have been described for foreign body removal. Some may occasionally be indicated, but all have significantly greater risks than removal with rigid endoscopy. Removal of esophageal foreign bodies using a balloon catheter has been described. This is a temptingly simple approach because it avoids the need for general anesthesia. However, there is a risk of esophageal perforation. The risk of airway obstruction is even greater because there is no control over where the foreign body will go after it is pulled from the esophagus. The risk of aspiration can be decreased, but not eliminated, by positioning the patient head down. Flexible endoscopy avoids the need for general anesthesia but does not afford as much object control as rigid endoscopy. Only small, flexible forceps can be passed through the instrument of a flexible scope. A rigid endoscope permits the use of a wide range of sizes and types of forceps, often specialized for a particular foreign body. For example, some forceps are designed to close safety pins prior to removal. Standard "alligator" forceps are not satisfactory for grasping round objects, such as beans or peanuts, and frequently propel such objects distally rather than grasping them. Specially curved forceps conform to the shape of peanuts. When using a rigid endoscope, the foreign body can often be pulled out through the lumen of the scope, so the patient is not subjected to further trauma from the object.

The use of meat tenderizer to dissolve impacted meat is extremely hazardous, as surrounding tissue is also digested. This technique should *never* be used.

When to Refer

Foreign bodies in the airway and those lodged in the esophagus or pharynx should always be removed, preferably with rigid endoscopy. Specialty consultation is indicated whenever this diagnosis is considered. For airway foreign bodies, the patient should be seen by an otolaryngologist, pulmonologist, and/or other surgeon experienced in the use of endoscopy to remove foreign bodies. An otolaryngologist, gastroenterologist, and/or other rigid endoscopist should be involved with pharyngeal and esophageal foreign bodies. Flexible endoscopy is sometimes indicated for diagnosis, and occasionally small foreign bodies may be effectively removed by this approach. However, rigid endoscopy is usually the preferred approach. If there is a possibility of esophageal perforation or a hazardous object beyond the esophagus, participation by a general surgeon in the removal of the object is mandatory.

KEY POINTS

— Esophageal foreign bodies in adults are usually impacted food, but in children, small objects are most common.

— Bronchial foreign bodies are usually encountered in children and are most often foreign objects or age-inappropriate food.

— A foreign body should be suspected when dysphagia or dyspnea occurs suddenly during eating or after an episode of coughing or choking.

— The classic triad of symptoms of bronchial foreign body (coughing, wheezing, and decreased breath sounds) are not present in all patients.

— Rigid endoscopy is the preferred technique for removing foreign bodies from the aerodigestive tract.

Suggested Readings

Darrow DH, Holinger LD. Foreign bodies of the larynx, trachea and bronchi. In Blueston C, Stool S (eds.): *Pediatric Otolaryngology.* Philadelphia: WB Saunders, 1996, pp 1390–1401.

Litovitz T, Schmitz G. Ingestion of cylindrical and button batteries: An analysis of 2382 cases. *Pediatrics* 89:747–757, 1992.

Ritter F. Questionable methods of foreign body treatment. *Ann Otol Rhinol Laryngol* 83:729, 1994.

Index

Note: Page numbers in *italics* refer to illustrations; page numbers followed by t refer to tables.

ISBN 0-7216-7431-3

90038